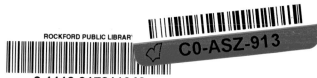
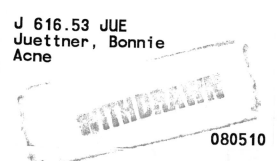
ROCKFORD PUBLIC LIBRARY

Rockford, Illinois

www.rockfordpubliclibrary.org

815-965-9511

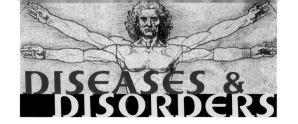

Acne

Titles in the Diseases and Disorders series include:

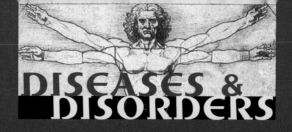

DISEASES & DISORDERS

Acne

Bonnie Juettner

LUCENT BOOKS
A part of Gale, Cengage Learning

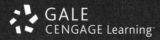

GALE
CENGAGE Learning™

Detroit • New York • San Francisco • New Haven, Conn • Waterville, Maine • London

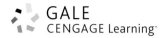

GALE
CENGAGE Learning

LIBRARY OF CONGRESS CATALOGING-IN-PUBLICATION DATA

Juettner, Bonnie.
  Acne / by Bonnie Juettner.
     p. cm. -- (Diseases and disorders)
  Includes bibliographical references and index.
  ISBN 978-1-4205-0215-2 (hardcover)
  1. Acne--Popular works. I. Title.
  RL131.J84 2010
  616.5'3--dc22

                                              2009033484

Lucent Books
27500 Drake Rd.
Farmington Hills, MI 48331

ISBN-13: 978-1-4205-0215-2
ISBN-10: 1-4205-0215-8

Printed in the United States of America
1 2 3 4 5 6 7 13 12 11 10 09

Printed by Bang Printing, Brainerd, MN, 1st Ptg., 12/2009

Table of Contents

"The Most Difficult Puzzles Ever Devised"

Charles Best, one of the pioneers in the search for a cure for diabetes, once explained what it is about medical research that intrigued him so. "It's not just the gratification of knowing one is helping people," he confided, "although that probably is a more heroic and selfless motivation. Those feelings may enter in, but truly, what I find best is the feeling of going toe to toe with nature, of trying to solve the most difficult puzzles ever devised. The answers are there somewhere, those keys that will solve the puzzle and make the patient well. But how will those keys be found?"

Since the dawn of civilization, nothing has so puzzled people—and often frightened them, as well—as the onset of illness in a body or mind that had seemed healthy before. A seizure, the inability of a heart to pump, the sudden deterioration of muscle tone in a small child—being unable to reverse such conditions or even to understand why they occur was unspeakably frustrating to healers. Even before there were names for such conditions, even before they were understood at all, each was a reminder of how complex the human body was, and how vulnerable.

While our grappling with understanding diseases has been frustrating at times, it has also provided some of humankind's most heroic accomplishments. Alexander Fleming's accidental discovery in 1928 of a mold that could be turned into penicillin has resulted in the saving of untold millions of lives. The isolation of the enzyme insulin has reversed what was once a death sentence for anyone with diabetes. There have been great strides in combating conditions for which there is not yet a cure, too. Medicines can help AIDS patients live longer, diagnostic tools such as mammography and ultrasounds can help doctors find tumors while they are treatable, and laser surgery techniques have made the most intricate, minute operations routine.

This "toe-to-toe" competition with diseases and disorders is even more remarkable when seen in a historical continuum. An astonishing amount of progress has been made in a very short time. Just two hundred years ago, the existence of germs as a cause of some diseases was unknown. In fact, it was less than 150 years ago that a British surgeon named Joseph Lister had difficulty persuading his fellow doctors that washing their hands before delivering a baby might increase the chances of a healthy delivery (especially if they had just attended to a diseased patient)!

Each book in Lucent's Diseases and Disorders series explores a disease or disorder and the knowledge that has been accumulated (or discarded) by doctors through the years. Each book also examines the tools used for pinpointing a diagnosis, as well as the various means that are used to treat or cure a disease. Finally, new ideas are presented—techniques or medicines that may be on the horizon.

Frustration and disappointment are still part of medicine, for not every disease or condition can be cured or prevented. But the limitations of knowledge are being pushed outward constantly; the "most difficult puzzles ever devised" are finding challengers every day.

A Common Problem

"**P**eople expect you to walk around looking like you do in the magazines," complains model Naomi Campbell. "Everyone has zits. I don't care if the whole world sees."[1] Campbell is just one of a long list of celebrities who struggle with acne. The list includes Kate Moss, Cameron Diaz, Britney Spears, Leonardo DiCaprio, Brad Pitt, Keira Knightley, Will Smith, Renée Zellweger, Tom Cruise, Elizabeth Hurley, Nicolas Cage . . . the list goes on and on, and it runs the gamut from teenagers to older people. Unlike Campbell, actress Knightley says she does care if the world sees her skin when she has a breakout. "Airbrushing is sort of nice because I always get acne," she says. "So . . . when they take it out digitally—I wish they could do that in my everyday life."[2]

It is not surprising that famous actors, actresses, and models experience acne. According to dermatologists, acne is a nearly universal condition. Dermatologists estimate that between 40 and 50 million Americans suffer from acne, including 80 percent of those between the ages of fifteen and thirty. Acne is the most common skin disease in the United States, more common than dandruff, athlete's foot, eczema, warts, or skin tags. "Almost all adults experience some form of acne," explains Vail Reese, a San Francisco dermatologist and movie buff whose hobby is running a Web site, Skinema, devoted to analyzing the skin of actors and actresses. He continues:

"These flares range from the rare deep cyst and closed pore to severe inflamed nodules. Acne lesions can be painful or itchy, and recurrent crops can be embarrassing and depressing. Fortunately there are a multitude of treatments for acne."[3]

Teenage Acne

Although most adults have periodic acne flare-ups, teens usually have more pimples per square inch of skin than adults do, according to Reese. Most acne sufferers first experience

Studies show that nearly 100 percent of teenagers between the ages of twelve and seventeen have acne at least occasionally.

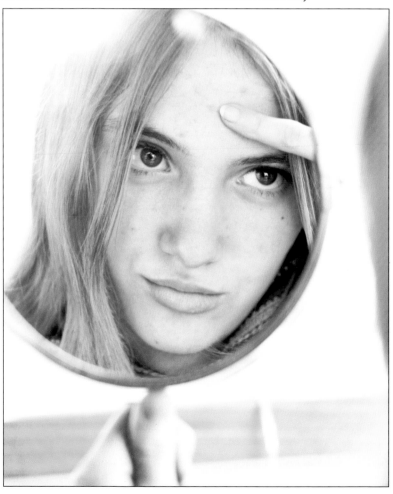

breakouts when they are teenagers. According to the American Academy of Dermatology, almost 100 percent of teenagers between the ages of twelve and seventeen have acne at least occasionally. The Centers for Disease Control reports that when preteens are included in the statistics, 80 percent have acne. In teens and preteens acne is triggered by the hormones that the body begins to produce at puberty. Race and ethnic background make no difference. Sex, though, does make a difference. Boys tend to have worse acne breakouts than girls do, because male hormones have a stronger effect on the sebaceous glands of the skin—the glands that produce oil. Both sexes, though, find acne breakouts to be extremely stressful.

"I guess it really hit when I turned sixteen," remembers one acne sufferer. "It even got so bad that when I had my senior pictures taken and I saw the proofs, I got sick. . . . I left school, sat in my car, and cried. I would not let anyone see them, not even my family. It wasn't until I had them retouched that I ended up showing them to anybody."[4]

Adult Acne

Although boys tend to have worse breakouts than girls as teenagers, in adulthood the trend reverses itself. Women are much more likely than men to develop acne. About 25 percent of men and 50 percent of women have acne as adults. In adulthood, as in the teenage years, acne is made worse by hormones, and women experience more hormonal events than men do—menstruation, pregnancy, menopause. Women may even find that their acne gets worse during adulthood than it was during the teenage years. Some women who had perfect skin in adolescence develop an acne problem in their twenties or thirties.

"I would say ninety percent of my patients that are women say the same thing," says Paul Jarrod Frank, a dermatologist who specializes in cosmetic conditions. "'I never had it as a teenager and why now?' Most importantly they want a reason and a cure. Hormonal fluctuations. Teenagers go through bouts of hormonal fluctuations but because of women's natural cycle it prolongs."[5]

Acne and Self-Esteem

Like other body conditions that are affected by hormones—weight, height, and sexual development, for example—the state of a person's skin can affect how that person feels about him- or herself. Living with acne can be hard on a patient's self-esteem. Teenagers, especially, may view a lesion as more noticeable than it really is—a pimple that others do not see may appear enormous to the eyes of an adolescent scrutinizing his or her appearance in the mirror. "I would have done anything to make it go away,"[6] remembers Paula Begoun, whose acne was not cured until she was in her twenties.

Although acne itself is not serious, psychologists say that about 50 percent of teenagers with acne develop psychological conditions stemming from it. Sandra Osborne remembered how her fifteen-year-old son, Sterling, reacted to his breakouts. "He is good-looking, but when the acne got bad he would say 'Why would anyone want to go out with me?'" she recalls. "His confidence was low."[7] Teens with acne often have increased levels of social anxiety, low self-esteem, and depression.

Adults with acne frequently also have a hard time feeling confident in social situations. "When I was in a professional environment," reports Alicia Garnes, now a stay-at-home mother living in Denver, "it felt like I was hard to take seriously."[8] Journalist Jess Weiner used to feel the same way. "The blemish becomes magnified, at least in your own mind. It impedes you from feeling sexy, or fresh, or clean."[9] Weiner covered her acne with makeup for years. Then one day she decided to go without her trademark concealer—and no one seemed to notice the difference. The acne, she realized, was far more visible to her than it was to anyone else.

"I have a vision," says *San Francisco Chronicle* columnist Mark Morford. Morford says he wants to start a magazine that will have one rule: no Photoshopping, no airbrushing—no digital enhancement of photographs whatsoever. People in the magazine, even celebrities, would look the way they would look if one met them on the street. "There will be pimples," he writes. "There will be blemishes. There will be wrinkles and scars and flab and sag, stretch marks and cigarette burns and age spots. . . . Won't that be wonderful? Won't that be refreshing?"[10]

Like the media, people with acne tend to take one of two possible approaches to their skin. They can try to "Photoshop" or "airbrush" it themselves—by putting on layers of makeup. During most of the twentieth century, women dealt with acne in this way. They wore concealer on specific spots and added a layer of foundation over the whole face. "What happens is that you sit for two and a half hours in front of the mirror covering up your imperfections,"[11] says Campbell.

But in the twenty-first century, in many parts of the country, the natural look came back into style. Women wear less makeup and often try to look as though they are not wearing any makeup at all. It is becoming more acceptable to take Morford's approach to skin problems—wash and dry the skin, leave it alone, and look the way humans really look. If enough people with acne take this approach, it may be possible to redefine beauty. Beauty does not have to mean smooth skin. Instead, it could mean kindness, compassion, grace, and wisdom—qualities that reside on the inside, not the outside, of the human skin.

CHAPTER ONE

What Happens During an Acne Breakout?

Many people with acne report that how a breakout makes them feel is more devastating than how a breakout makes them look. "I felt tortured," says Paula Begoun when she recalls the acne breakouts she had in her twenties. Like many acne sufferers, she dreaded looking in the mirror in the morning. "Every morning it was a sense of 'Okay, what's it going to be?' when I looked in the mirror."[12]

Fifteen-year-old Andrew Murray felt the same way. He would look in the mirror and assess what people would think when they first saw him. "It bothers me because your face is usually the first part of your body that people notice, and when you have acne, it makes you feel awkward,"[13] he says.

Diagnosing Acne

As Begoun and Murray can attest, acne is easy to spot. It does not ordinarily take a doctor to recognize it. Most acne sufferers diagnose their condition for the first time themselves, at home.

Acne can develop almost anywhere on the skin. It usually appears on the face, chest, shoulders, or back. Its location tends to vary depending on a person's age. But acne sufferers often find it most distressing when they discover new blemishes on their faces. In teenagers acne usually crops up on the forehead, nose, or chin. Adult women tend to get acne on their chins and around their mouths. Elderly people develop whiteheads and black-heads on their upper cheeks and on the skin around their eyes. Wherever it develops, acne tends to cause redness and swelling. It may also produce pain, itching, or tenderness of the skin.

The Body's Largest Organ

Although people do not see acne in the mirror until it reaches the surface of the skin, acne breakouts are only the outer man-ifestation of a process that begins deep under the skin's sur-face. The skin is the body's largest organ. It consists of three layers: the epidermis, dermis, and subcutaneous tissue. The epidermis is the outer layer, the surface where acne becomes visible. The dermis is a thicker layer, housing a network of nerve endings, blood vessels, hair follicles, and sweat and se-baceous, or oil, glands. Under the dermis lies the subcutaneous tissue, which includes a layer of fat that insulates the body and cushions it from bumps and falls. Altogether, the skin makes up about 15 percent of a person's body mass. It is the main or-gan in the integumentary system, which also includes the hair, nails, and sebaceous and sweat glands of the dermis. (Not everything in the dermis is part of the integumentary system. For example, nerve endings are part of the nervous system, and blood vessels are part of the circulatory system.)

The skin covers and protects the body's internal organs, but it also does much more than that. It helps the body to maintain homeostasis. This means that the skin helps the body to stay in balance by helping it maintain a healthy temperature and by excreting substances that the body needs to get rid of. The skin removes water, salt, and waste substances, such as urea, from the bloodstream, and the sweat glands excrete them in sweat. (Most urea is excreted in urine, but a small amount is excreted in sweat.) At the same time, the body's sebaceous glands ex-crete oil, the body's natural moisturizer. This oil lubricates the skin and protects it from germs.

The Sebaceous Glands

The skin's sebaceous glands and sweat glands are located in the skin's deep inner layer, called the dermis. Each person has

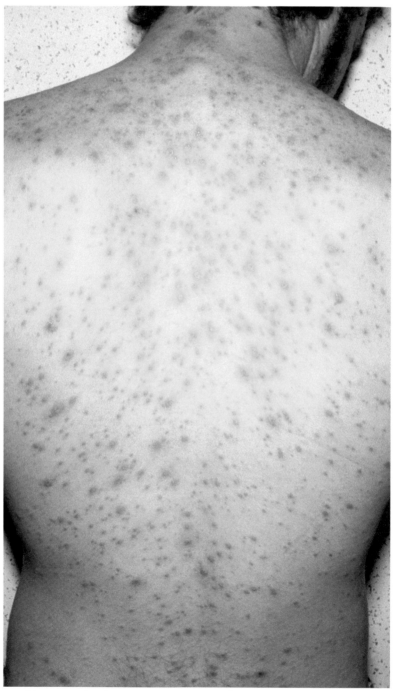

In addition to the face, acne can appear almost anywhere on the skin.

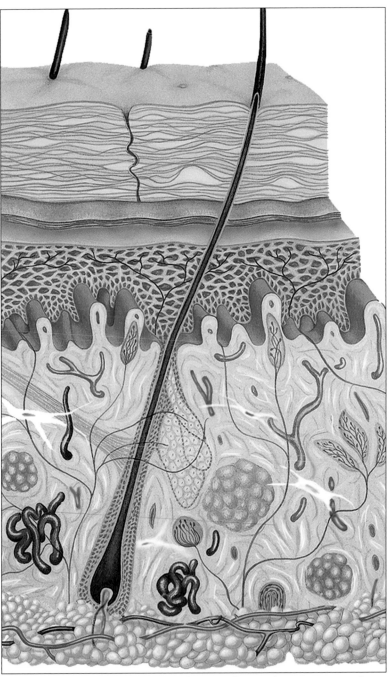

The skin consists of three layers of tissue: the epidermis, or outer layer; the dermis; and the hypodermis, or subcutaneous fat.

between 2 million and 5 million glands—more than ten glands for every square millimeter of skin. The sebaceous glands are located within hair follicles, small sacs in the skin out of which hairs grow. Each hair follicle is lined with cells from the epidermis, the skin's outer layer. The sebaceous glands open out into the follicles, providing sebum to moisturize the hair as it grows. There are hair follicles all over the body, not just on the head, because tiny, fine hairs, called vellus hairs, grow all over the body, even on the face, chest, and back.

Acne begins in the sebaceous glands. Because there is such an extensive network of sebaceous glands throughout the skin, it is possible for a person with acne to develop a fairly extensive and severe case of the condition. Acne usually begins when the sebaceous glands suddenly start to increase the amount of oil, or sebum, that they produce. Sebum production increases at puberty and during other hormonal events such as menstruation and menopause. The extra sebum sometimes causes dead epidermal skin cells to stick together, forming a plug that dermatologists call a comedo. The resulting blemish is then called a comedone.

Doctors do not know why acne forms in particular hair follicles and not others. "To me, one of the most incredible mysteries is how come only some follicles are involved at any given time," remarks Pennsylvania dermatologist Albert Kligman. "You've got thousands of sebaceous follicles on your face. . . . But maybe you've only got ten or fifteen or twenty comedones. Here's one follicle with a comedo, and right next door, here's one that's normal. Why is that? Whatever it is, we simply don't know."[14]

Blackheads and Whiteheads

Superficial cases of acne are mild and stay close to the surface of the skin. The comedo blocks the opening of one of the skin's pores. If the pore is closed, the blocked pore is called a whitehead. If the pore is open, the melanin, or pigment, in the comedo reacts chemically with oxygen in the air. It causes the comedo to darken, so this kind of blocked pore is called a blackhead. In blackheads and whiteheads, there is no redness,

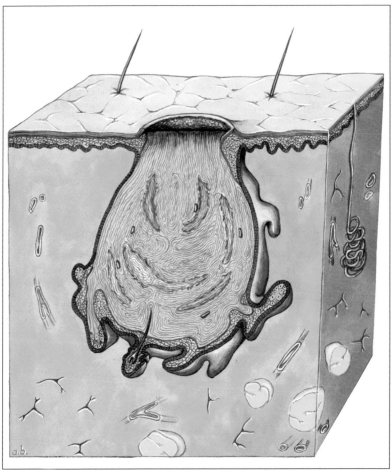

Sebum production causes dead epidermal skin cells to stick together and form a comedone, or blackhead.

or inflammation, so blackheads and whiteheads are considered noninflammatory acne.

For people with mild cases of acne, the acne may consist only of blackheads and whiteheads. In moderate or severe cases, though, acne continues to progress and the blackhead or whitehead becomes infected and inflamed. The infection is caused by *Propionibacterium acnes* (*P. acnes*), a bacterium that normally lives deep in the skin. An infected blemish will turn red and begin to swell in size. At this point it is called a pimple.

Once a pimple has become infected, it is no longer considered a whitehead or a blackhead. Instead, it gets a different name, depending on its appearance and location. A small, firm, red bump is called a papule. It does not contain any obvious pus and is located relatively near the surface of the skin. A papule that is full of obvious pus is called a pustule. The pus in a pustule tends to be white and gooey. It is made up of white blood cells. A pustule that is located deep under the surface of the skin is called a nodule. Nodules are also called cysts. They can be tender and painful, and they take a long time to heal.

Dermatologists classify acne according to whether it consists mostly of whiteheads and blackheads or whether it tends to produce cysts. People who get only a few blemishes at a time and who tend to get mostly whiteheads and blackheads

---

Acne-Like Conditions

Dermatologists used to consider any skin condition erupting out of the sebaceous glands to be acne. But in recent years, some conditions have been reclassified. Doctors have found that hair follicles can be irritated by cosmetics, allergic reactions to chemicals, or mechanical irritation such as clothing rubbing against the skin. When irritated the skin may break out in blemishes that look like acne pimples but technically are not, since they are caused by contact with an irritant rather than by dead skin blocking a pore. This kind of acne-like condition is called an acneiform eruption.

Another condition that can be mistaken for acne is the appearance of milia, which are often called "milk bumps" because they are common in newborns. Milia are tiny bumps that look much like whiteheads. Like acne, milia are caused by dead skin blocking pores, but they are not connected with an overproduction of sebum. Milia bumps do not swell up and become red and inflamed like a pimple. Instead, they look like tiny, white bumps just below the surface of the skin.

are said to have mild acne. People who sometimes get cysts and who tend to have more frequent lesions have moderate acne. And people who get mostly cystic acne and who get many lesions at any given time have severe acne.

Acne's Side Effects

Acne is not a physically serious or life-threatening condition, but it can upset the people who have it. Acne has two side effects that tend to disturb its sufferers. First, it can be painful and itchy. Second, people with acne tend to view their skin as unsightly, and the appearance of acne on their skin can lead to anxiety, low self-esteem, and depression. Even after acne lesions clear up, they can leave scars that mar the appearance of the skin.

Any condition that causes skin inflammation in the form of redness and swollen tissues can be physically uncomfortable. The skin is packed full of nerve endings. One kind of nerve ending, called a mechanoreceptor, detects touch. Mechanoreceptors on the surface of the skin detect light touch, and those deeper in the skin detect hard pressure. Some mechanoreceptors are connected to hair follicles, where acne forms. Another kind of nerve ending, pain receptors, detect chemicals that are released when cells in the skin are damaged. The skin has some pain receptors that detect sharp pain, such as a pin prick, and other pain receptors that detect blunt or throbbing pain, such as the pain of a bruise. The redness, or inflammation, caused by swollen, red pimples or cysts below the skin can activate the skin's pain receptors, resulting in tenderness, itching, or pain.

Scarring

Inflammatory acne can do more than cause tenderness and pain. Once it heals it may also leave a scar. Two types of scars are common in acne patients. In the most common type of scar, skin tissue has been lost. The healed pimple leaves behind a pit, or hole, in the skin. In the other kind of scar, skin tissue has been added as the skin heals. The new tissue creates a raised bump on the skin.

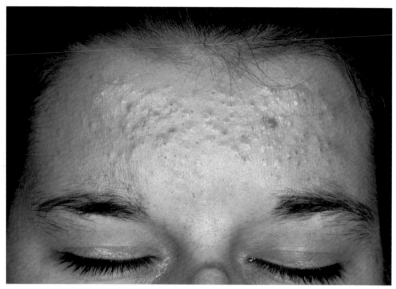

This woman's forehead has been scarred by acne.

Acne may also leave behind a mark that looks like a scar but is actually a change in the skin's pigment. These marks are neither raised nor pitted but look like spots on the skin. Doctors call these spots hyperpigmented macules, and the skin's tendency to form them is called postinflammatory hyperpigmentation. *Hyper* is a prefix meaning "above normal," and *pigment* refers to the skin's melanin, the substance that gives skin its color. A macule is a discolored spot, like a freckle. (Melanin also causes the changing color of skin that is tanning in the sun.) *Postinflammatory* means "after inflammation," or after redness and swelling occur. So with postinflammatory hyperpigmentation, there is more pigmentation than normal occurring in a place that was recently inflamed. Hyperpigmented macules form because inflamed skin releases more melanin than usual. The melanin is trapped in place by white blood cells. In skin that is pale, the extra melanin may appear as a red or pink spot. In skin that is darker, the spots may appear to be much darker than the surrounding skin. Macules left by acne are not permanent, but they may last for months or years after the original blemish has faded.

Even when acne does not leave a scar or a macule, it leaves an irregularity in the skin. A hair follicle that has been stretched out and inflamed will always be slightly distorted. It will not return to its original size or shape. This kind of skin irregularity is not visible in itself to the naked eye, but when there are a lot of irregularities in acne-prone skin, they can give the skin a motley, rough appearance.

Psychological Effects of Acne

Even when acne greatly changes the appearance of the skin, doctors tend to think of it as a trivial condition, one that may not even need to be treated. Acne is not life-threatening and does not make it harder to function physically on a day-to-day basis. But studies show that, especially for teenagers, acne can be associated with psychological problems, including depression and anxiety. "Whoever thinks acne is no big deal has never had any," says actress Vanessa Williams. "You're stared at, you're judged, and if you're a kid, you're even picked on."[15]

Even a mild case of acne, such as the appearance of one pimple a month, may be upsetting to teenagers, who are at an age when young people tend to be obsessed with how they look. "Acne teaches us to look for flaws," says Gail Robinson, former president of the American Counseling Association. "That becomes habitual, a way of viewing yourself."[16] One American Medical Association study showed that teens with acne have lower self-confidence and tend not to participate in social activities that they might otherwise enjoy. One college student remarked: "The only good thing about my acne is I'm getting great grades, because when my skin is broken out I just sit in my apartment and study. It's so sad, but that's the way I feel. I just don't go out."[17]

Even celebrities with acne find that it affects how they feel about themselves. Tennis star Serena Williams says that acne lowered her self-esteem and made her want to stop playing tennis. "If I'm worrying about my skin, I'm distracted and can't play my best," she says. "It's like having a big spotlight on your face. I felt like 'Oh, God, I'm gonna be on the court and playing in front of millions of people worldwide. Is that photographer gonna snap this volcano on my right cheek?'"[18]

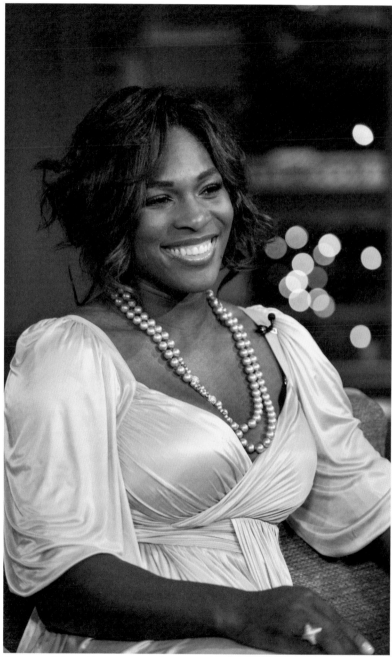

Even acclaimed international tennis champion Serena Williams admitted that acne breakouts lowered her self-esteem and affected her game.

Acne and Suicide

Psychologists think that acne is driving some teens to suicide. It is hard to be certain that acne is the cause, however, because teenagers, as a group, are very prone to depression and suicide. Suicide is the third most common cause of death for teenagers. In 2007, 15 percent of U.S. teenagers said they had considered suicide in the preceding year. Seven percent said they had actually attempted it. It is likely that many of those teenagers suffered from acne, but was acne the cause of the suicides?

Researchers say that in some cases, the answer may be yes. A 2001 study showed that 40 percent of acne patients (teens and adults) experienced clinical depression, low self-esteem, and suicidal thoughts as a result of the acne. And a 2006 study showed that nearly one-third of teens with severe acne think about killing themselves. In the 2006 study, 10 percent told researchers they had actually tried to kill themselves. About 24 percent said the acne made them depressed, while 9 percent reported anxiety related to acne. These teens may not have realized that acne is treatable or that celebrities who appear to have perfect skin in magazines or in video footage have usually had their images airbrushed or digitally altered.

Another woman who had severe acne as a young adult remembered: "When I was in college I was out on a date with this guy who said, 'you know, you'd be really attractive if you didn't have such bad acne.' I banned the word 'acne' from my house after I got married. My husband couldn't say 'acne' or 'zit,' the only thing he could say was 'blemish' if he had to say anything at all, because it brought up such terrible memories."[19]

Even though people with acne may feel as though they are the only ones who look the way they do, statistics show that acne is a nearly universal experience. Imagine that researchers decided to stop ten people at a random location such as a bus stop and ask each person if they had ever had acne and if so, how they felt about it. Statistically, it is likely that at least nine out of those ten people (if they were all over the age of twelve) would say that yes, they had had acne at some point, and no, they did not like how it made their skin look. Fortunately, acne can be treated as well as covered up with makeup. The first step in treating acne is to figure out its cause.

CHAPTER TWO

Causes of Acne

"**A**s a teenager, I'd break out a lot," says Jennifer Berry. "I would get one or two really big blemishes, on my forehead, or my cheeks and chin, and they'd last forever. . . . I felt like no matter how much makeup I put on, that's all people looked at."[20]

When Berry turned seventeen she began competing in the Miss Oklahoma pageant. The stress made her breakouts even worse.

> Pageants are funny because you're trying to be at your best, but it's a very stressful time leading up to the final night. You wear more makeup than usual, practice hard for the talent show, stay up late, get up early. You just feel like your face is falling apart.
>
> I competed in the Miss Oklahoma program five years in a row and . . . it was the same every time. As the week progressed, my skin started breaking out. It would get worse and worse and worse.[21]

Berry began to hope that she would not win the pageant, because she was afraid to have the photographs show all her breakouts. Eventually, though, she was able to treat her skin, and her acne cleared up. She became Miss Oklahoma 2005 and Miss America 2006.

Teenage Hormones

Berry's acne followed the same pattern that most people experience. She began to develop acne as a teenager and stress made her acne worse. Actress Chrishell Stause had a similar experience: "I first started having acne problems in eighth grade, when I was about 14. All of a sudden I went from this

The pituitary gland is shown in this computer illustration. The gland stimulates the release of estrogen in females and testosterone in males.

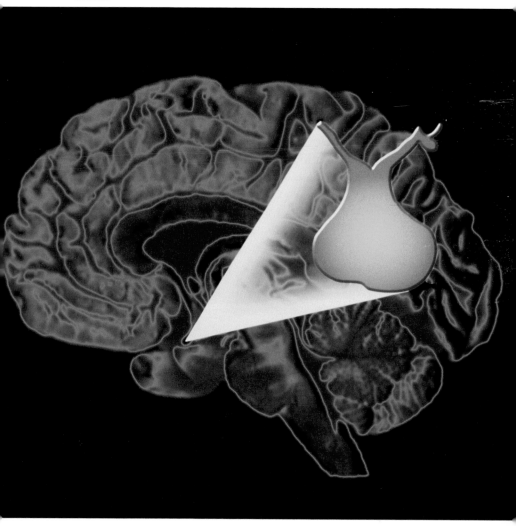

perfect little kid face to a nightmare of tiny bumps all over my forehead."[22]

Acne is most common after puberty. It is thought that nearly all teenagers experience acne, whether it is mild, moderate, or severe, at some point. During puberty, two glands in the brain, the hypothalamus and the pituitary gland, release hormones that have a dramatic effect on the body, including the skin. Glands are a type of organ, just as the heart, lung, kidneys, and even the skin itself are organs. The hypothalamus and pituitary glands are located in the brain, but other glands are located throughout the body.

Certain glands, rather than having their own function, exist for the purpose of regulating the work of other organs. They do this by releasing hormones—chemicals that tell different organs in the body what to do. Glands operate throughout a person's life, not just during puberty. For example, the thymus, a gland in the chest, responds to infections. It releases hormones that stimulate white blood cells to mature. The adrenal glands, located just above each kidney, release hormones during times of stress. These hormones make a person more alert and increase breathing and heart rates.

During puberty, the hypothalamus and the pituitary glands stimulate the body to grow and develop. They release hormones that stimulate the ovaries in girls to release estrogen and the testes in boys to release testosterone. They also stimulate the ovaries and adrenal glands to produce small amounts of testosterone in girls, and they stimulate the production of small amounts of estrogen in boys. Scientists are not sure why, but in both boys and girls, testosterone and other androgens, or male sex hormones, can stimulate the sebaceous glands to produce more sebum. Boys produce about ten times more testosterone than girls do, so boys are much more likely to develop acne as teenagers.

The sebaceous glands are sensitive to testosterone and other hormones that are classified as androgens for a reason. The skin cells, hair follicles, and sebaceous glands contain androgen receptors—places that can easily bind with androgens in the bloodstream. Androgens do a lot of good for the skin. They help the skin cells to grow and divide so that skin can replace itself more quickly. They also help hair to grow and become thick. (Men have more body hair than women because androgens bind with androgen receptors in their skin and cause more hair to grow.) Even stimulating the sebaceous glands is good for the skin in some ways, because the sebum that is produced moisturizes the skin and protects it. However, when the sebaceous glands are stimulated too much, they can produce too much sebum—and acne is the result.

Adult Acne

After teenagers the second largest group of acne sufferers is adult women. For some women adult acne is just a continuation of the acne that they experienced during their teenage years. Many women, however, do not experience acne as teenagers and experience it for the first time when they are in their twenties. The acne of adult women, like that of teenagers, is usually caused by hormones. "When adult women experience acne outbreaks, hormones are usually the primary culprit,"[23] says Diane Berson, who teaches dermatology at Weill Medical College of Cornell University in New York. The hormone surges that adult women have are similar to those of teenage girls and are caused by the glands that regulate women's monthly menstrual cycle.

Like teenagers some adult women find it embarrassing to connect their acne with their monthly periods. "Women . . . were using euphemisms like 'stress bumps' or 'monthly breakouts' to describe their problems," observes Katie Rodan, a San Francisco dermatologist. "They thought acne was an ugly four-letter word or they thought acne was just for teenagers." Rodan explains that monthly breakouts are a form of acne. "It is not a curable problem, but it is treatable and manageable,"[24] she says. Berson agrees but notes that adult women may need the help of a dermatologist to treat their acne. "Hormonal acne can be particularly frustrating because it may not respond to the same over-the-counter treatments that worked for some women during their teenage years,"[25] she says.

Polycystic Ovary Syndrome

Sometimes acne turns out to be just one symptom of an under-lying disorder. Adult women who have severe acne may need to be evaluated for polycystic ovary syndrome, especially if they are obese and have thinning hair. They may even develop other symptoms, such as hair growth on the face, chest, stomach, thumbs, or toes. They may also have some pelvic pain and patches of thick or dark skin. In polycystic ovary syndrome, the ovaries, and sometimes the adrenal glands, produce a higher-than-normal level of androgens. The extra androgen interferes with the development and release of eggs by the ovaries. As a re-sult, fluid-filled sacs or cysts can develop on the ovaries. That is why the syndrome is called polycystic.

Women with polycystic ovary syndrome may be infertile. Most of the time, their ovaries do not release eggs for fertiliza-tion. Instead, the ovarian follicles that hold the eggs bunch to-gether and form cysts on the sides of the ovaries. The eggs remain in the cysts and are not released. This means that it can be very difficult to get pregnant. It can also cause women to have very irregular menstrual cycles. They may not have normal men-strual periods at all.

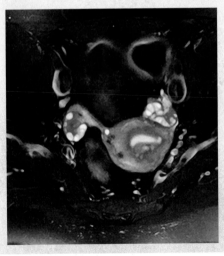

Women with polycys-tic ovary syndrome can be treated with medication. Often they also see im-provement in their symp-toms if they lose weight.

A magnetic resonance image (MRI) shows polycystic ovarian cysts (in white) forming on the ovaries (green).

Pregnancy and Menopause

Puberty and menstruation are not the only physical events that can cause hormonal disruptions in a woman's body. During pregnancy and menopause, many women experience acne flare-ups. Pregnancy affects different women differently. For some women the large levels of estrogen circulating through their bodies during

During pregnancy many women experience outbursts of acne due to high levels of the hormone progesterone.

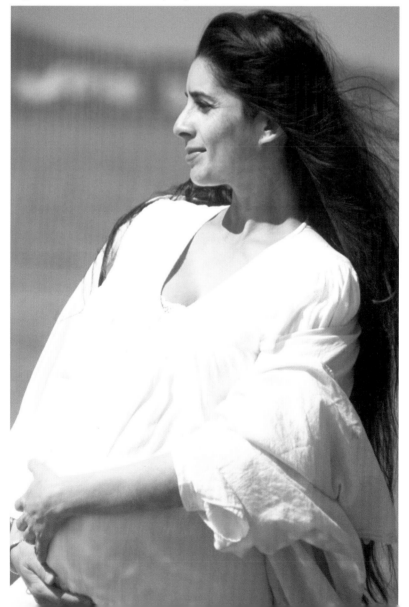

pregnancy suppresses androgens, and their skin clears up. Other women, though, find themselves reacting to the high levels of progesterone that are produced in pregnancy. After ovulation progesterone levels begin to climb. Progesterone is chemically related to testosterone. It can have the same effect on sebaceous glands that testosterone does, increasing the production of sebum and leading to more acne.

During menopause, on the other hand, estrogen levels fall dramatically, but testosterone levels remain about the same. Since estrogen suppresses the androgen receptors in the skin, the testosterone that previously did not affect the sebaceous glands may suddenly start to stimulate them, leading to an increase in sebum production. As a result, women going through menopause may also experience acne flares.

Stress

Many people with acne think that their breakouts are not caused by hormones, but by a different factor: stress. Actress Jennifer Love Hewitt feels that her acne was brought on by stress. "I was really stressed out and tired," she says. Hewitt developed cystic acne, deep under the surface of her skin. "Obviously I'd used concealer here and makeup there to try to cover it up," she goes on, "but that's difficult stuff to cover. . . . When they put me in *Maxim* as one of the sexiest women in the world, they had to airbrush my photo because I had pimples on my face."[26] Singer and actress Jessica Simpson had a similar experience with acne around her chin and mouth, as she explains:

> I was on my first tour, and the stress was just amazing. I had a terrible, terrible breakout. I just started looking sad because of the blemishes that I had. And when I shot my videos, they had to go in and digitally fix my chin. It was to the point where I was embarrassed to go onstage or do photo shoots . . . my fans . . . were just shocked when they saw me. I wasn't what they saw on the cover of the magazine.[27]

Dermatologists agree that stress can cause acne. But stress is not unrelated to the body's hormone levels. Stress dramatically affects the functioning of the hypothalamus and pituitary glands in the brain. Stress also affects members of both sexes by stimulating the adrenal glands to release two other hormones: adrenaline and cortisol. These hormones can make the skin more susceptible to acne in two ways. First, when adrenaline is released, so are androgens. These androgens, like testosterone, can bind with the androgen receptors on the sebaceous glands and stimulate the production of more sebum.

Adrenaline and cortisol also suppress the body's immune system. The body becomes less able to fight off infection, so bacteria are more likely to succeed in infecting comedones. The body also becomes slower at healing wounds, so acne lesions heal more slowly than they otherwise would.

In 2007 researchers became interested in the effect of stress hormones on acne. They tracked the changing skin of ninety-four high school students. They also monitored students' stress levels. During periods when emotions were running high and there was a lot of pressure, like the week before major exams, students were 23 percent more likely to have acne breakouts. In this study, though, students' sebum levels did not change—but their comedones became infected, red, and inflamed much more easily than they did at less stressful times.

Psychologist Ted Grossbart of Harvard Medical School says that patients who think their acne might be caused by stress should ask themselves several questions. Does the acne get worse during times when they are very emotional? Does it get better when there is less stress? Is the acne harder to treat than the doctor or dermatologist thinks it should be? Do symptoms get better or worse in a way that seems random or erratic? If there is no other reason for the acne and it tends to be associated with stress or it changes at random, there might be a psychological cause. A psychological cause is even more likely if the patient is someone who tends to appear stoical and calm at stressful times. In those cases, psychologists hypothesize that the patient might appear calm, but still be holding a lot of stress internally. Only the patient, however, can say whether or not this is really the case.

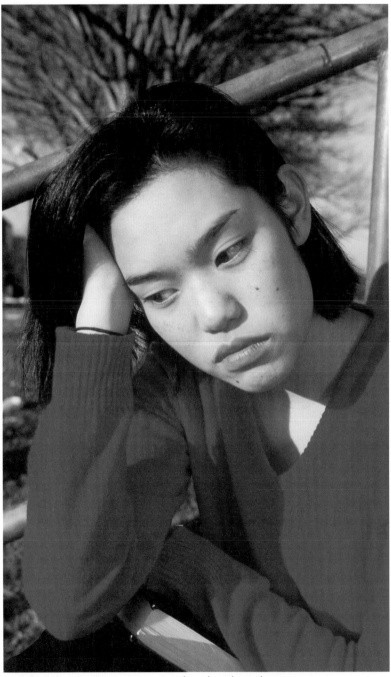

Some teens experience acne outbreaks when their emotions are running high or they are distressed over something.

The Skin's Ecosystem

Once hormone levels increase, whether they do so because of puberty, pregnancy, stress, or for some other reason, sebum levels go up as well. By increasing sebum and by slowing the body's ability to repair its own tissue, hormones set into motion a series of events that can lead to the formation of comedones. Before acne can become red and swollen, though, something else has to happen—the comedone must be infected by the bacterium *P. acnes*. But *P. acnes* is present in the skin of almost all people, not just acne sufferers. Except at birth, human skin is not sterile, even after it has been washed.

Measuring Sebum

Sometimes dermatologists need to measure the amount of sebum that a patient is producing. Collecting sebum, though, is a challenge. Over the years, dermatologists have come up with several creative methods. The oldest method is to press cigarette paper against the forehead for three hours, and then analyze the sebum on the paper. Another method is to use a cold, frosted glass plate. When the glass plate is pressed against the skin, sebum on the skin's surface seeps into microscopic pockets in the surface of the glass. Later, doctors can light up the glass and study the pattern of light scattering. The pattern shows which areas of skin have the highest concentration of sebum.

Recently, many doctors have begun using a tool called Sebutape, an adhesive tape. First, they apply bentonite gel to the patient's forehead, leaving it there for twelve to twenty-four hours. The bentonite gel soaks up and depletes the excess sebum stored in reservoirs in the skin. Once the excess sebum is removed, Sebutape is applied to the forehead. Sebutape is white, but it turns clear when sebum is absorbed. After three hours the Sebutape is removed. It is placed on a black background. Then dermatologists can see the pattern as a series of black dots (the places where the tape turned clear) on a white background.

In fact, the average human not only has *P. acnes* in his or her skin, but a host of other microbial residents as well. A normal human typically has as many bacteria and yeasts living on the surface of the skin as there are people on earth. Viruses and mites live on the skin's surface too.

Usually, having a variety of microorganisms living on the skin helps the body to stay healthy. For example, the skin's resident bacteria get in the way of other organisms that might want to invade the skin. Bacteria also break down substances that the skin secretes, or gives off. These secretions may be released by the sebaceous glands, the sweat glands, or the apocrine glands (specialized sweat glands in the armpits and groin). Sometimes, though, the population of organisms living on the skin can become unbalanced.

The bacterium *P. acnes* is one kind of organism whose population in the skin can become unbalanced. *P. acnes* can survive and thrive only in places where there is no oxygen. It lives deep in the skin, where it feeds on sebum. When hormones cause the sebaceous glands to produce more than the usual amount of sebum, it is easy for *P. acnes* populations to swell. Applying antimicrobial gels and creams to the surface of the skin may not do any good, because *P. acnes* is not located at the surface. As bacterial populations get out of control, the body's immune system responds. White blood cells flock to the area to fight the bacteria. At this point, the comedone, or blemish, may begin to swell, turn red, and feel tender and warm.

Although *P. acnes* can get out of control, in 2009 researchers discovered that people who have a large and diverse population of bacteria on their skin are less likely to develop acne. Scientists at the National Human Genome Research Institute hypothesize that a healthy person should have around 112,000 different species of bacteria living in and on the skin. While examining the skin of volunteers, they found that oily skin has fewer species of bacteria living on it than dry or moist skin does. One theory is that *P. acnes* gets out of balance when it does not have enough other bacteria to compete with it.

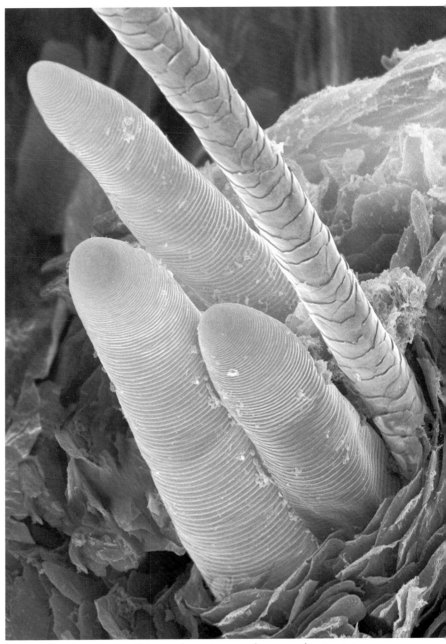

The microscopic tails of *Demodex* mites can be seen digging into an eyebrow hair. According to some dermatologists, mites can cause problems, such as acne, if the mites living in a person's hair increase and break out of the hair follicle.

Mites

Bacteria are not the only skin-dwelling organism that can cause acne. *Demodex* mites live in the hair follicles of most people. Between 96 and 98 percent of humans have *Demodex* living in their hair, where the mites feed on oils, hormones that are excreted by glands in the scalp, and fluids around the hair follicles. "Many people don't like the idea of bugs living in their hair and on their skin, and some get really bent out of shape just thinking about it," says Jerry Butler, a University of Florida professor of entomology. "For some folks, it's enough to make [their] skin crawl. And bathing won't wash them off."[28]

Although people may not like the thought of mites living in their hair, *Demodex* mites are harmless, unless their population begins to increase suddenly. "When something causes the mites to reproduce at a higher rate," says Butler, "they can break out of the hair follicle and may cause acne, hair loss, and skin conditions. In some cases the interaction with mites causes skin to actually slough off."[29] Not all dermatologists agree that mites can cause problems. Frank Flowers, a professor of dermatology at the University of Florida's Health Science Center, argues, "No skin disease in humans has been conclusively linked with these mites."[30]

Genes

Some acne is thought to be genetic. People are most likely to get it if one of their parents had it. If both parents had it, "the gun is pointed directly at you,"[31] says Food and Drug Administration (FDA) dermatologist Carnot Evans. Researchers studying the human genome are beginning to hunt for the gene or genes that make a person more likely to develop acne. A genetic tendency to develop acne could affect a person in various ways. A person might have a genetic tendency to produce more androgens or might simply be more sensitive to them. Or a person might have a genetic tendency to heal slowly from wounds or to become infected easily.

Even if the cause of acne is genetic, it can still be treated. Understanding why a patient is especially susceptible to acne is important, because it can affect the choice of treatment. Hormonal imbalances may be treated one way, while bacterial infections are treated differently. If the cause of acne is something temporary, such as puberty or pregnancy, a person might decide not to treat it but just to live with it for a while. People who suffer from severe acne, though, usually decide to try to treat it. In the end they may go to a dermatologist. But at first they usually try to treat the acne themselves.

CHAPTER THREE

Self-Treatment of Acne

Most acne sufferers treat their acne themselves, using home remedies or over-the-counter creams from a drugstore. Only about 7 percent of teenagers with acne ever see a dermatologist. Even fewer adults do. About 80 percent of acne is never seen by a dermatologist.

Sunlight

Many people begin their self-treatment of acne by spending more time outside, getting lots of fresh air and sunlight. This is an optimistic approach, which probably only works for mild, easily resolved cases of acne. It is true that sunlight and fresh air will kill bacteria and that bacterial infections can make acne more severe. Some people find that their acne improves in the summer, when they can spend a lot of time in the sun. But *P. acnes*, the bacterium associated with acne, is located deep within the skin, not at the surface. And some doctors feel that sunlight stimulates the sebaceous glands. "In my practice, the busiest time of year for acne is October," says New York dermatologist Laurie Polis. "People go out in the sun in the summer; the sunlight stimulates the follicles. And a few months later, you've got more acne."[32]

Dermatologist Carnot Evans of the FDA thinks that sunlight may help, but not directly. Instead, it may help by reducing

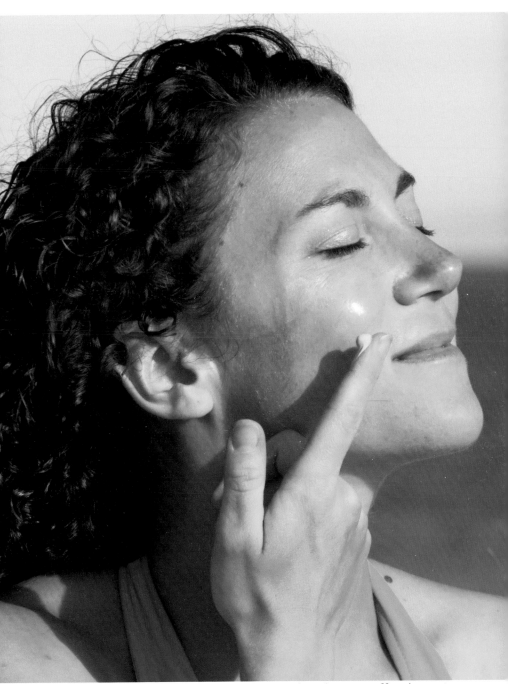

Sunlight kills some acne-causing bacteria but does not affect bacteria that live deep under the skin.

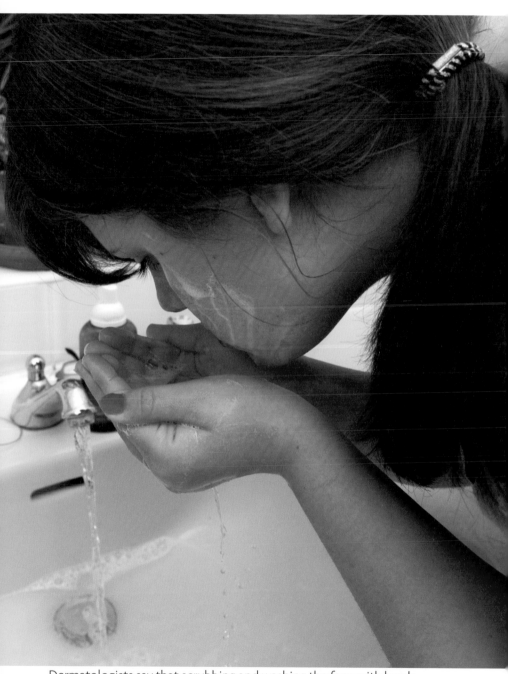

Dermatologists say that scrubbing and washing the face with harsh cleansers can irritate the skin and break down its defenses, resulting in more acne.

stress—giving people an opportunity to relax outside. "It's hard to say whether it's the sun or the psyche that has an effect on acne," he comments. "The sun may have a modest effect in some people, but the relaxation usually associated with summer is also probably a factor."[33] Warm summer weather may also encourage people to spend more time exercising, which also reduces stress.

Washing and Scrubbing

Sunlight and fresh air alone are unlikely to cure a case of acne. Another self-treatment that acne patients often turn to is cleaning the skin more often and more severely. Many react to new breakouts by scrubbing their skin clean several times a day with harsh cleansers. Dermatologists caution that this is probably one of the worst things one can do. "Acne is rarely the result of poor hygiene," says Yardley, Pennsylvania, dermatologist Richard Fried. "Attempts to clean or even sterilize the skin often cause more problems than they solve."[34]

Fried explains that too much scrubbing and sterilizing can irritate the skin. "Aggressive cleaning in general is one of the worst mistakes people can make," agrees doctor Susan Bershad. "Overly aggressive cleansing causes skin swelling. And when you have skin swelling, it tightens the pores, trapping stuff in the lower portion of the follicle. And that can make the acne even worse."[35]

Even normal skin that is not especially acne prone can develop lesions in response to repeated scrubbings. Scrubbing the skin very hard, using abrasive cleansers, or applying strong chemicals can cause the skin's normal defenses against foreign invasion to break down. Overly vigorous cleansing can allow irritants and allergens to enter the skin. In some cases scrubbing can result in an infection by bacteria, viruses, or fungi. As a result, the skin is likely to become red and angry looking.

"Most people want to get rid of their acne yesterday," says dermatologist Marianne O'Donoghue. "So they go out and buy Oxy 10, and maybe cleansing grains to wash with, and maybe an astringent with alcohol, and before you know it, their faces are like raw meat."[36] Scrubs that contain rough abrasive elements, like pieces of walnut, are especially bad for the skin, she says. "Years ago, when I first started practicing, we used to use these really abrasive cleansers—like apricot scrubs," she remembers. "But then all these patients started coming in with calcium deposits below the surface of the skin. The particles got into the pores, and the skin reacted just like an oyster making a pearl!"[37]

Being Gentle with Sensitive Skin

People with acne tend to have sensitive skin that is especially easily irritated. Sensitive skin may be able to tolerate even less washing and scrubbing than normal skin. "Scrubs tend to be harsh," says beautician Shalea Walker. "If you have acne, a scrub can cause your skin's bacteria to travel."[38] Walker tells her clients to use a gentle cleanser and a moisturizer. Dermatologist Diane Berson agrees. However, she also recommends that, at least during the premenstrual week for women, patients use a toner containing salicylic acid or glycolic acid, which may help remove surface oil from the skin.

The gentlest cleansers, Walker feels, are those made out of mechanically engineered microbeads. Although acne-prone skin should not be scrubbed with harsh soaps, gentle soaps that are used should be kept on the face for at least two minutes, not rinsed off right away. "What most people do with cleansers is just rinse them off right away," says dermatologist Alan Shalita. "We say lather up and keep it on for a couple of minutes." This is especially true if the cleanser contains medication to prevent acne from forming. "Salicylic acid . . . penetrates fairly quickly, so if you leave it on for a few minutes it does the trick,"[39] says Shalita.

O'Donoghue recommends that her patients simply not use soaps that contain medication. Soaps with acne medication in them, she feels, can be too harsh. She warns:

> If you are using a benzoyl peroxide or salicylic acid soap all over your face, that area under the eye where the skin is so thin and tender can get really sore and irritated. I would rather see a patient use Dove on her whole face

Squeezing Pimples

Squeezing a pimple to empty it of its pus is a common reaction. Unfortunately, dermatologists say that squeezing or picking at a pimple is unlikely to help. Instead, it may lead to a bacterial infection. A pimple that becomes infected on its own is likely to be infected by *P. acnes* bacteria. But a pimple that is picked open and squeezed may be colonized by bacteria that live on the surface of the skin, such as strep or staph. Most people have staph bacteria living on their skin or in colonies under their fingernails, so it is easy to accidentally introduce those bacteria into an open pimple while squeezing it.

When a pimple becomes infected with staph, it is likely to get worse, not better. The infection may, like a *P. acnes* infection, cause redness and swelling. In addition, because the pimple was picked open, it may have a scab. It will take longer to heal, is more unsightly, and is more likely to leave a scar than it would have if it had been left to heal on its own.

Dermatologists recommend not popping a pimple because it could lead to infection.

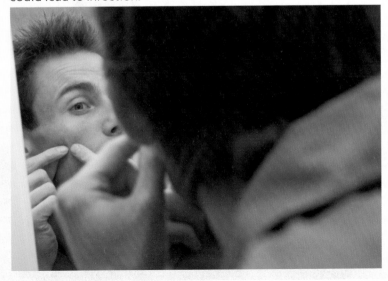

and then put the acne medicines just where she needs them. Also, while it may be okay to use an acne soap with an over the counter acne lotion, if you are using an acne soap with a prescription acne treatment, you can end up being chapped and unable to use the prescription where you need it.[40]

Moisturizer and Sun Protection

Walker advises her clients to moisturize their skin as well as wash it. She advises each client to have two moisturizers on hand—one for days when skin tends to be oily and one for dry days. Most people, she says, find that their skin is different on different days. "I try to get people to realize the differences in their skin," she says. "Your cheeks don't do the same thing as your forehead. Your skin doesn't do the same thing every day."[41] Although some people believe they have dry skin, Walker says that they may actually have dehydrated skin. Dehydrated skin may be more easily irritated than normal skin, but it can easily be hydrated by using moisturizer and drinking plenty of fluids.

Just as important as moisturizing skin, according to dermatologists, is protecting it from the sun. Berson explains, "Daily sun protection is essential as some acne medications increase the skin's sensitivity to sunlight."[42] Even if acne sufferers are not using medication on their faces, sunscreen can prevent damage to the skin from the ultraviolet radiation in sunlight.

"Also, when buying cosmetics or other skin or hair care products," Berson continues, "look for ones labeled noncomedogenic —meaning they do not clog pores and are less likely to cause acne."[43] A noncomedogenic product is one that does not tend to cause the formation of comedones. Some makeup can cause an acneiform eruption—an outbreak of spots that look like acne but are not technically acne, since they are not caused by an overproduction of sebum. These spots are called acne cosmetica. If spots appear overnight, though, they are not acne cosmetica, but a different condition: chemical folliculitis. Folliculitis occurs when follicles in the skin become red, inflamed, and

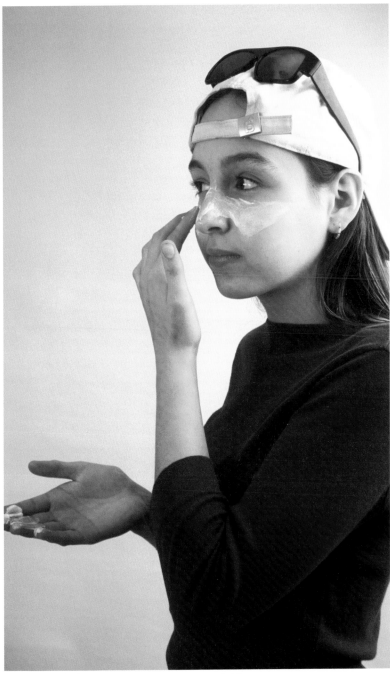

For teens, daily sun protection is essential because some acne medications increase the skin's sensitivity to sunlight.

irritated. When folliculitis is caused by a reaction to chemicals, such as the chemicals in cosmetics, it is called chemical folliculitis. When chemical folliculitis develops, the cure is to stop using the product that produced the reaction.

Over-the-Counter Remedies

If ordinary washing and moisturizing does not improve a case of acne, the next step is usually to try an over-the-counter remedy —a remedy that people can buy for themselves without a prescription. Dermatologists say that over-the-counter remedies can work quite well for people who have mild acne—acne that consists mostly of whiteheads and blackheads and is located at or near the surface of the skin. "They don't work as fast as prescription medicine. Or as effectively," cautions Shalita. "But they do work. If you've got mild acne—a few pimples, a couple of comedones—you may never have to go beyond the drugstore."[44]

The two most commonly used ingredients in over-the-counter acne medicines are benzoyl peroxide and salicylic acid. Both benzoyl peroxide and salicylic acid will dissolve in oil, which means they can penetrate deep into the skin—if they were unable to dissolve in oil, the oil in the sebaceous glands

When to Stop

Over-the-counter remedies containing benzoyl peroxide and salicylic acid are considered safe for consumers to use without first consulting a doctor. But patients should stop using benzoyl peroxide if it causes an increase in redness, produces an itching or burning sensation or a rash, or causes blisters to form. Symptoms like this may be a sign of an allergic reaction. Users should also wash their hands after applying benzoyl peroxide—it has a whitening effect and may bleach clothing, sheets, or towels. It should not lighten the skin, but it may lighten hair if it is applied near the hairline.

would form an impenetrable barrier that would keep them out. However, these two drugs act in different ways; they are not interchangeable.

Benzoyl peroxide is commonly prescribed by dermatologists because it is an antibacterial. It will kill *P. acnes* bacteria. But it is not necessary to get it from a dermatologist. "You can get the same amount of benzoyl peroxide at a drug store at a fraction of the cost and it will work as well, provided that you use it,"[45] says dermatology professor Hilary Baldwin, who teaches at the State University of New York.

Salicylic acid, on the other hand, is an exfoliant and an anti-inflammatory agent. As an exfoliant, it can loosen the comedones that get stuck in hair follicles, helping to release the comedones from the skin before they can cause a plug. For this reason, it is helpful for preventing acne. Once a plug is formed, salicylic acid's anti-inflammatory properties may be helpful because it can reduce redness and swelling. But it will not remove all large comedones, and it may take several months to dislodge small ones from the pores in which they are stuck.

Acne sufferers looking for a product that contains benzoyl peroxide or salicylic acid have a plethora to choose from. It is important to choose a formulation that is right for one's own skin. Most teenagers do well with ordinary benzoyl peroxide. As teenagers reach the age of about nineteen or twenty, however, they may want to make a change. Young men may find that their acne clears up at around that age, while young women may need to transition to different products. "A lot of products . . . geared to teens are too drying for older skin," says Bershad. "Women use them, and their skin gets irritated, and then they go and use moisturizers that are really heavy, and that makes their acne worse."[46]

Bershad advises young adult women, in particular, to use both benzoyl peroxide and salicylic acid, but to use them separately. One product could be used at night and one in the morning. Or, she says, patients should at least wait twenty minutes between applying different products. Otherwise, it is possible that a chemical reaction between the benzoyl peroxide and the salicylic acid could inactivate some of the salicylic acid's ingredients. People who use over-the-counter remedies should also be especially careful to be gentle when they wash their skin. Skin that has been scrubbed until it is raw is likely to be even more irritated by benzoyl peroxide or salicylic acid.

Preventing Acne

According to dermatologists, no treatment is very effective for pimples that have already formed. While dermatologists recognize that some over-the-counter products claim to get rid of acne that has already formed, they are skeptical. The key to treating acne, they say, is to prevent it from occurring in the first place. "Acne treatment is preventative, not something you use to get rid of the pimples you've already got,"[47] says Shalita. "Once you have a blemish, it's really too late," agrees Bershad. "Acne treatments don't cure zits, and they are not meant to."[48]

Over-the-counter remedies are effective for preventing acne from forming. This means that when an acne sufferer begins using an over-the-counter remedy, he or she should not expect immediate results. The remedy should reduce inflammation and help to prevent new pimples from forming. The already existing pimples must heal on their own, over the course of time. This process can take six to eight weeks for pimples and deep cysts. Blackheads and whiteheads may take even longer—up to three months.

Living with Acne

Because it takes so long for acne to heal, people with acne have no choice but to live with it, at least for a short period of time. Some acne sufferers choose to live with it permanently. They reason that acne is not a life-threatening condition, and it can be easily concealed with makeup. Atlanta dermatologist Jodi Ganz agrees with this approach. "One piddling little zit is not going to hurt you, it is not contagious and you might not need to do anything to treat it," she argues. "At the same time, you do worry about people with severe acne who might waste a year and hundreds of dollars trying something that is not going to work for them."[49]

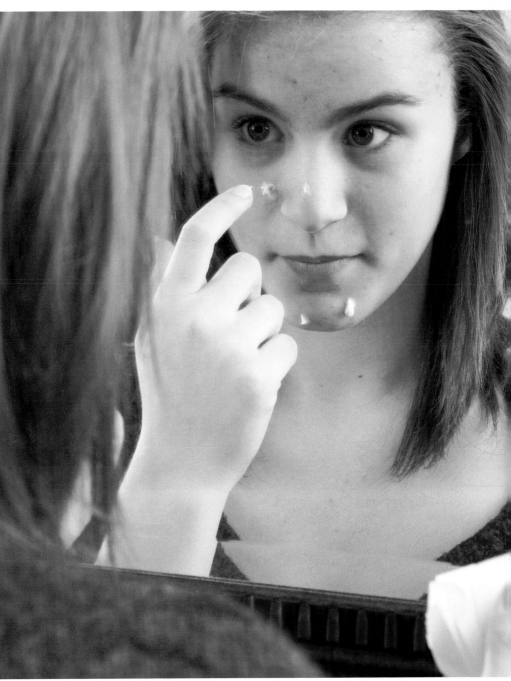

Although over-the-counter acne products containing benzoyl peroxide are effective, they take time to work.

Treating acne at home with over-the-counter remedies or simply choosing to live with it both work well for people who have mild cases of acne. It is a good option for people who only have occasional acne flare-ups or whose acne does not tend to get red and inflamed. For people with moderate or severe acne, though, self-care may not be enough. Severe acne, especially acne that consists of deep cysts and nodules under the skin, may not clear up without medical care. For teens and adults who have this kind of acne, the next step is to visit a dermatologist.

CHAPTER FOUR

Medical Treatment for Acne

When Irish actor Keith Duffy was a teenager he stayed at home behind closed doors as much as possible. The kids at school called him names because of his acne. "At 14 or 15 I got an awful time at school. Some mornings my face was so bad my mother wouldn't even send me to school," he remembers. "Brunch, Pizza-Face, Join-the-Dots: I got all the names."[50]

When to See a Doctor

Many teenagers react to acne just the way that Duffy did. When acne first begins, they try to treat it themselves, and they avoid going out when they do not have to. But over-the-counter remedies can be expensive, especially if they do not work. Avoiding social engagements can be hard on a teen's self-esteem, and skipping school can be hard on a teen's academic record. When self-treatment and over-the-counter creams do not help, it may be time to see a doctor. "It's a personal choice," says Kent Taulbee, a Bloomington, Illinois, dermatologist. "We see people at all stages. I think if it's becoming a problem socially, you're worried about long-term scarring and it's interfering with your lifestyle and self-esteem, it's time to see me."[51]

People with acne should also see a dermatologist if they are not sure whether the condition they have is acne or something else. Eruptions that look like acne pimples may actually be

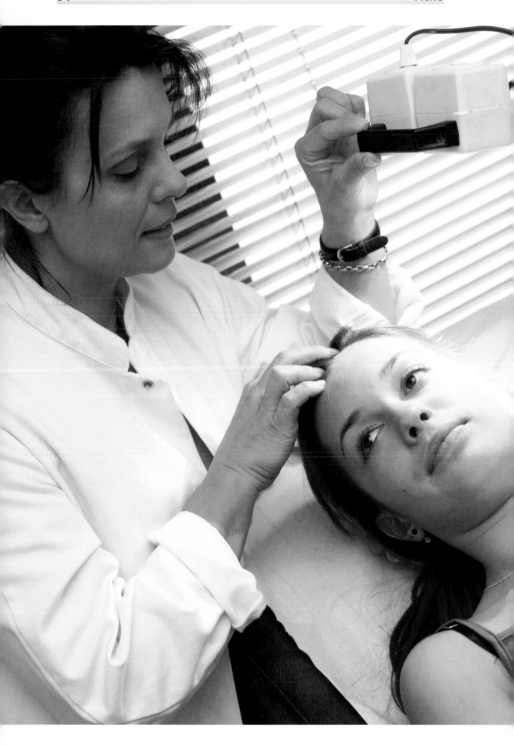

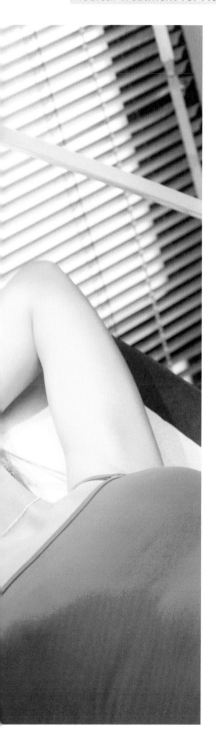

rosacea, contact dermatitis (a reaction to a new cosmetic, lotion, or piece of clothing), or in rare cases, even skin cancer. It is also important to see a specialist if acne appears in an unusual location, such as an armpit. And people who know that they have other skin disorders (like rosacea, dermatitis, eczema, or skin cancer) should discuss their acne with a dermatologist, because treating two skin conditions simultaneously can be tricky.

A dermatologist will begin the diagnosis of acne in much the same way an acne sufferer would at home—by looking at the skin in good light. Dermatologists can check to see if the acne is deep or just on the surface, if it is infected, and whether or not there is scarring or skin discoloration. In some cases a dermatologist will order a blood test in order to rule out another disorder. In rare cases a dermatologist might order a stool test, if he or she suspects that bacterial overgrowth in the intestines might be contributing to the disease.

Once the diagnosis of acne has been confirmed, the next step is to identify the cause and treat it. Dermatologists can treat acne at any point in its development—by attacking the bacteria that can cause an infection, by opening the pores and reducing the likelihood

Some acne sufferers will only go to a doctor or dermatologist after they have exhausted over-the-counter acne remedies.

that a comedone will form and plug a hair follicle, or by trying to adjust the balance of hormones in the body that can cause sebum production to increase in the first place.

Antibiotics

In one of his most difficult cases, Fried suspected that the acne was caused by a bacterial overgrowth. When dermatologists

---

Antibiotic Resistance

Doctors are beginning to rely less on antibiotic drugs for treating bacterial infections, because many bacteria have evolved into strains that can resist the most commonly prescribed antibiotics. When bacteria are exposed to a drug that kills them, most of the bacteria causing the infection will die. But a few mutant bacteria may survive. The mutant bacteria, by chance, evolved characteristics that made them able to survive the drug. Mutant bacteria evolve all the time, but they do not normally become dominant, because they do not reproduce any faster than ordinary bacteria. But when an antibiotic kills all the other bacteria, mutant bacteria have a chance to reproduce in greater numbers—they do not have to compete with other bacteria. Since bacteria reproduce every few hours, a strain of antibiotic-resistant bacteria can quickly evolve and entrench itself in the body. Antibiotic resistance is even more likely to develop when doctors prescribe a broad-spectrum antibiotic, one that targets a wide variety of bacteria.

Dermatologists use a narrow-spectrum antibiotic, one that only targets *P. acnes*, to treat patients with acne. Because the antibiotic used to treat *P. acnes* is more narrow, doctors originally thought that it would be less likely to lead to antibiotic resistance. However, now dermatologists estimate that as many as 60 percent of acne patients have acne caused by an antibiotic-resistant strain of *P. acnes*. This means that antibiotics are becoming less and less effective as a method for treating acne. Antibiotics can help some patients, but not others.

suspect that acne is being caused by an overgrowth of bacteria, they often prescribe an antibiotic, a drug that kills bacteria. Antibiotics can be taken orally, or they can be applied to the acne in the form of a cream. (Most over-the-counter acne creams also contain ingredients such as benzoyl peroxide that are meant to kill bacteria.) In the case of his patient Susan, Fried prescribed both. He says: "I asked that she abandon (at least temporarily) her over-the-counter products and use only the products I recommended. I prescribed a brief course of antibiotics combined with topical medications. The regimen was clear and simple, and it allowed Susan to wear whatever makeup she desired. Her skin responded quickly."[52]

Not only did Susan's acne improve, but over time, it went away entirely. It is not usually a good idea for an acne patient to stay on antibiotics forever, though. "I believe that you should always be looking for an exit strategy,"[53] says Fried. He was able to convince Susan to take steps to reduce her stress levels. She began to spend less time working and more time pursuing her social life and hobbies, and she was able to discontinue her antibiotic treatment.

Why is it so important for Susan and other acne patients to minimize the amount of time they spend taking antibiotic drugs? Antibiotics have side effects, including increasing a person's sensitivity to the sun and upsetting the gastrointestinal tract. Antibiotics kill bacteria, but the body relies on its bacterial balance to stay well. People on antibiotics are more at risk for yeast infections as a result. In addition, any time that a person takes antibiotics, there is a danger that antibiotic-resistant bacteria may evolve. Antibiotic-resistant bacteria are bacteria that cannot be killed with any of the commonly used antibiotics.

Retinoids

Not all acne is infected with bacteria, however. For some patients, antibiotic treatment does little good. For patients who have blackheads and whiteheads that do not tend to get infected, many dermatologists prefer to begin by prescribing a retinoid. Retinoids such as Retin-A, or tretinoin, are medicines that are derived from vitamin A. They work by reducing the formation of microcomedones—the little plugs of dead skin cells that block the pores and cause acne to develop—and by keeping the pores open. By stopping the formation of microcomedones, retinoids can prevent acne from forming. But they also treat acne that has already developed by reducing inflammation. This means that pimples and cysts that have already formed may start to shrink and may become less red. Because retinoids both prevent acne and treat current flare-ups, they can be very effective at clearing the skin. "This ingredient works better than anything else," says dermatology professor Joel Cohen of Retin-A. "It actually works to remodel skin on a cellular level."[54]

Retinoids have some side effects, however. The most common are dry skin and chapping. Retinoids can also cause redness and inflammation that is similar to a sunburn. The skin may also become very sensitive to sunlight. Patients who use retinoids must commit to using sunscreen regularly to protect their skin. "The medicines I tried really dried out my skin," commented actress Chrishell Stause after her first few visits to a dermatologist. "Sometimes it was painful and I became very sensitive to the sun. . . . The medicines basically took away one problem, but added more."[55]

Isotretinoin

Dermatologists say that one retinoid—isotretinoin, commonly known as Accutane—is the most powerful acne drug they have ever found. Dermatologist Richard Fried says that "for most people, it essentially 'fixes' acne, at least for a while."[56] It helps the cells inside hair follicles to become normal, reduces sebum production, and reduces inflammation—so cystic acne becomes less red and swollen. Since 1984, when isotretinoin first became available, about 12 million patients have used Accutane to defeat severe, persistent cystic acne.

Even though it is very effective, isotretinoin, like other acne treatments, takes about two months to make a difference. Patients may even continue to see their acne get worse for the first few weeks. Like other acne treatments, isotretinoin prevents future acne breakouts while giving existing breakouts a chance to heal on their own. Ordinarily, patients take isotretinoin for a period of about four months. This is enough to cure acne permanently for many patients. For others, the benefits of isotretinoin last for many years, but eventually the acne returns. A few patients also find that isotretinoin does not work in their particular cases.

Dermatologists have used the most powerful acne drug ever developed, Accutane, to defeat severe cystic acne.

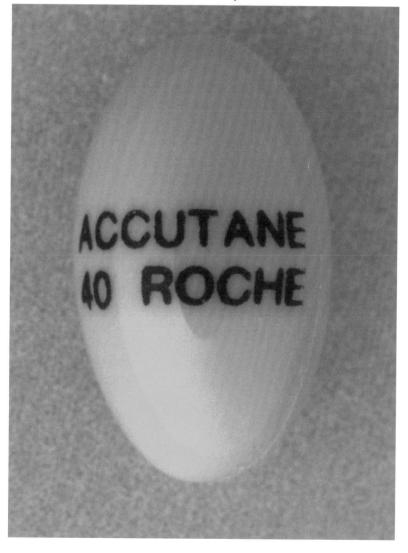

Birth Defects

Isotretinoin can be a miracle drug for many acne patients. However, isotretinoin is controversial because it also has some serious side effects. Isotretinoin is safe to take prior to conceiving a baby. But if a pregnant woman takes isotretinoin, even if she only takes a small amount for a short time, her fetus is likely to develop severe birth defects. The woman may even miscarry. The birth defects are likely to be especially severe if a woman takes isotretinoin in the first three months of pregnancy, a time period when she may not yet realize that she is pregnant. The baby may be blind, deaf, or mentally retarded, may have heart defects, or may have brain problems such as an unusually small brain or a brain in which the fluid-filled spaces are unusually large.

Before prescribing Accutane for a woman of childbearing age, dermatologists often insist that she take two pregnancy tests to make absolutely sure she is not pregnant. They also insist that women of childbearing age who take Accutane have a plan in place to avoid becoming pregnant, such as using contraception or abstaining from sex. Women who do not abstain from sex may be asked to use two forms of contraception simultaneously to be absolutely sure that they do not become pregnant. They may also be asked to take a monthly pregnancy test. Longtime acne sufferer Paula Begoun chose to abstain from sex with her husband while taking Accutane. Patients usually do not take Accutane indefinitely—they take it for around sixteen weeks. Begoun felt the weeks of abstinence were worth it. "I had tried everything, and nothing worked," she says. "I would have done anything, and I mean anything, to make it go away at that point."[57]

Isotretinoin and Depression

Birth defects are not the only serious side effect that has been connected with isotretinoin. Some researchers have associated isotretinoin with serious depression and an increased risk of suicide. Scientists began studying a possible connection between isotretinoin and suicide in 2002, after a fifteen-year-old flying student deliberately flew a small plane into the side of an office building in Tampa, Florida. The accident occurred during a psychotic episode that his mother said began after he started taking isotretinoin. The flying student was not the only teen to have a psychotic episode just after beginning a prescription of isotretinoin. Over the next several years, other isotretinoin users had psychotic episodes, too, and many dermatologists felt the link might be real.

However, two large studies in 2005 and 2009 showed no connection between isotretinoin and depression or suicide. There is, though, a link between having acne and becoming depressed or suicidal. Some scientists think that patients taking isotretinoin are slightly more likely to become suicidal in the first place, because they have severe acne. Psychiatry professor Madhulika Gupta, the author of the 2009 study, concluded that the truth lies somewhere in the middle—she felt that in some rare cases, isotretinoin does push certain patients over the edge. "Over the years," she writes, "I have seen a few patients who are on isotretinoin who became emotional, irritable, and sometimes suicidal. So, I have no doubt that some people do become suicidal, even some who had no previous psychiatric problems."[58] Gupta advised dermatologists not to shy away from prescribing isotretinoin, but to carefully monitor any patients who are taking it and to watch for possible changes in their mental states.

Despite the possibility of side effects, most acne patients who take isotretinoin are very happy with the results. Bonnie Estridge, who was struggling with acne caused by polycystic ovaries, says that she avoided taking the drug until she had tried every other possibility she could think of. "The whole idea of the drug scared me completely," she says. But her acne kept getting worse. During the first few weeks on isotretinoin, her acne continued to worsen. Then, gradually, it began to improve. "Everyone kept telling me I looked fantastic," Estridge reports. "It was hard for people to believe my skin had cleared up as it had. There were some scars left, but they could be covered easily with makeup. I could wear halter-necks, swimsuits, be proud to show off my body for the first time. I felt brilliant, bursting with confidence. Life was worth living."[59]

Oral Contraceptives

In some cases dermatologists prefer not to treat the skin conditions that occur after sebum production has gone up but instead to balance the hormones to which the sebaceous glands are so sensitive. This approach does not work with boys and men. But teenage girls and adult women with acne usually are reacting to hormones released during their bodies' monthly menstrual cycles. For most of the month, high estrogen levels may suppress sebum production caused by androgens. But just before a period begins, estrogen levels suddenly drop. That is when acne tends to flare up.

In adult women premenstrual acne tends to flare up on the sides of the face, the chin, and the neck. "Pimples move south with age," says dermatologist Katie Rodan. "They'll be fewer in number but bigger in size."[60] This kind of acne tends to be mild but persistent. Dermatologists often treat it by prescribing oral

Retinoids and the Aging Process

Retinoids—creams and oral medications that are derived from vitamin A—are one of the most commonly prescribed treatments for acne. The American Academy of Dermatology considers retinoids to be useful in treating all types of acne. Retinoids have many negative side effects. They can dry the skin, cause irritation and redness, or provoke an allergic reaction.

One side effect of retinoids though is welcomed by some adults. Retinoids cause an increase in collagen, a protein in the skin that makes it more pliable and resilient. By increasing the skin's collagen, retinoids cause skin to be less wrinkled. Retinoids also lighten age spots. Adults using retinoids find that their skin feels smoother. However, because retinoids make the skin more sensitive to drying and redness, people who use them must also use sunscreen.

contraceptives—hormones that are normally prescribed to prevent a woman from becoming pregnant. When dermatologists prescribe oral contraceptives (OCPs), they are hoping that the high levels of estrogen in the contraceptives will suppress sebum production all month. "Birth control pills are especially useful in women who have acne that is worse around their periods,"[61] says Stamford dermatologist Samuel Gettler.

Like antibiotics and retinoids, OCPs have side effects. One side effect is obvious—they prevent pregnancy, so they are not appropriate for women who are trying to get pregnant. In addition, they are not safe for women who have hypertension, blood clots, or who are smokers over the age of thirty-five. "On the other hand," says Diane Berson, a professor at Weill Medical College of Cornell, "women taking OCPs may actually benefit from a decrease in developing osteoporosis and protection against endometrial and ovarian cancer. That's why it's important for women considering taking OCPs to discuss the pros and cons with their dermatologist."[62] Unfortunately, OCPs can be expensive, and insurance companies often refuse to pay for them.

Mechanical Treatments

While the cause of acne is being treated, most patients would like more than prevention of future outbreaks. They would like to have something done about the outbreaks they already have. But dermatologists say that it can take weeks or months to clear up pimples that have already formed. Most dermatologists prefer to start with a preventive approach, allowing pimples that have already formed to heal on their own and trying to stop new ones from forming.

It is possible for a dermatologist to drain existing cysts surgically or to extract the contents of whiteheads and blackheads through a process called comedo extraction. But comedo extraction can be painful and may leave scars. "I never do comedo extraction on the first visit," says dermatologist Alan Shalita. "Unless you want to antagonize the patient . . . extraction hurts."[63] Berson agrees, adding, "Never. You want to loosen them up first."[64]

To do a comedo extraction, a dermatologist uses a circular tool to press down gently all around the outside of the lesion, until the contents of the pimple have drained. If the comedone is closed, the doctor may use a surgical blade or needle to nick it open. The process is similar to what acne patients themselves may do if they pick at or squeeze pimples, but there is one big difference—a dermatologist can remove the contents of a pimple in a way that will not lead to infection and scarring. If the lesion is a deep enough cyst, a patient would not be able to drain it at home in any case. In those cases a dermatologist might inject the cyst with a corticosteroid to reduce inflammation and help the cyst to heal on its own.

Repairing Scars

It takes a long time to heal persistent acne. Once the acne is cleared up, patients are often left with scars that mar the surface of their skin. "I'm always crushed when patients come in with horrible acne scarring," says Miami dermatologist Alicia Barba. "It doesn't have to be that way."[65] Dermatologists do have some tools that they can use to improve the appearance of scars or, in some cases, to remove scars.

For mild acne scars the easiest solution may be to remove the top layer of skin. One option is a chemical peel. This involves a chemical solution, such as glycolic acid, trichloroacetic acid, salicylic acid, lactic acid, or carbolic acid. When applied to the skin, the chemicals in the solution damage the skin's top layers, causing them to separate and peel off. The new skin left after the peel is removed should be smoother and more even in color than the skin that was peeled off the surface.

A chemical peel is not done during the first office visit. Instead, patients may be given a cream to apply to the skin to prepare it for a peel. Then, when they return for the next office visit, the dermatologist begins by cleansing the skin to remove excess oil. Next the peel is applied. It usually feels warm or hot for about five minutes. There may also be some stinging.

Another option dermatologists sometimes use to remove the top layer of skin is dermabrasion. Instead of using chemicals, dermabrasion uses a rough substance to smooth away the top

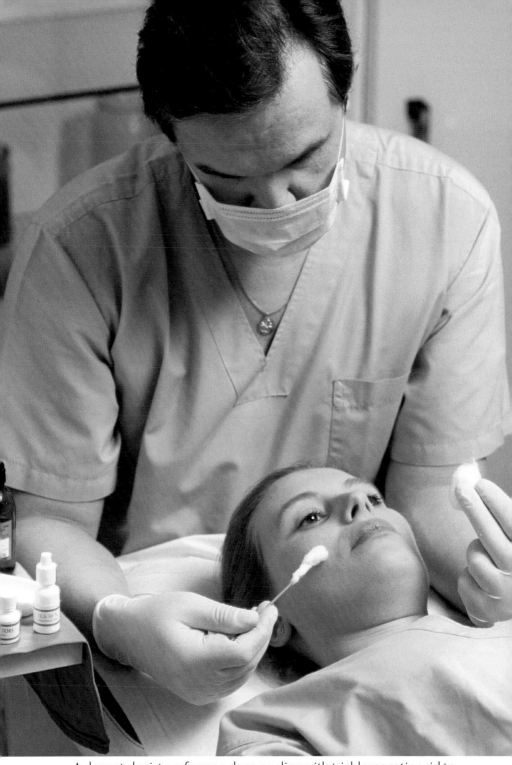

A dermatologist performs a deep peeling with trichloroacetic acid to repair acne scar tissue.

layer mechanically. It is like sanding the skin. Like chemical peels, dermabrasion damages the skin, and it can be painful. Afterward the skin may look and feel as though it has been badly sunburned. After dermabrasion, it takes about ten days for the skin to heal. At first the new skin is pink, but after two

A dermatologist uses an instrument to perform dermabrasion, a sanding of the skin, on a patient.

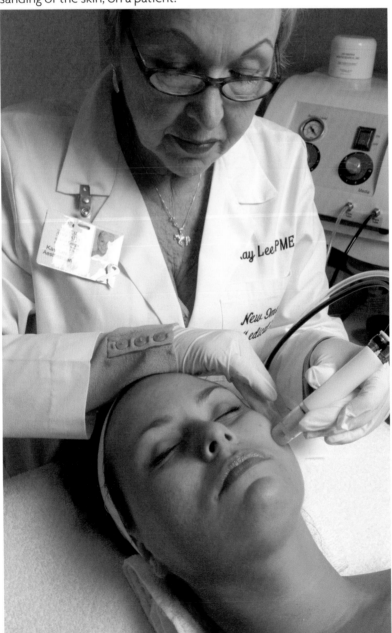

or three months, it looks like normal skin again. The old scars may not be gone, but their appearance and texture should improve.

For more serious scarring, dermatologists have other tools they can try. Some scars either leave a hole in the surface of the skin (this is sometimes called an "ice pick" scar) or leave extra material on top of the skin (a "box car" scar). To treat stubborn scars such as these, dermatologists sometimes excise, or cut away, the scar. They take away the smallest amount of skin necessary and sew the new wound shut neatly, hoping to replace a round, raised scar with a smooth, flat line. In severe cases, it is also possible to graft skin from another part of the body to fill the place where the scar was located.

Seeing Results

No matter what treatment acne patients seek for their condition, they have to be patient while waiting for the acne to improve. It takes time to find a treatment that is exactly right for each individual. Even the right treatment can take weeks to work, because acne takes weeks to form. The American Academy of Dermatologists says that it can take six months of treatment to get severe acne to clear up. "It often seems like an eternity before a breakout subsides and disappears," counsels Fried. "Keep in mind that each new breakout on your skin actually began forming about three weeks earlier."[66] Consequently, Fried says, it takes at least three weeks before a new acne treatment has a chance even to start to work. Barba agrees. "Be compliant and be patient," she counsels. "It can take months to see results. And it'll probably get worse before it gets better."[67]

CHAPTER FIVE

Alternative Treatments for Acne

Frank went to see dermatologist Richard Fried with stubborn acne that had lasted for more than four years. Frank had already been to several other dermatologists. He had found that he could keep about 80 percent of his acne at bay if he took high doses of antibiotics and used very irritating creams on the surface of his skin. But he could not heal the remaining 20 percent. He had even taken isotretinoin, or Accutane, but he was among the minority of patients who are not helped by it. Though Frank was skeptical, Fried decided to try an alternative approach with him.

Over the next several months, Fried convinced Frank that he should get enough sleep and try to reduce the amount of stress in his life. "Frank learned stress management techniques," remembers Fried. "He set a goal to listen to a guided imagery relaxation tape for ten minutes at bedtime. He also made a conscious effort to better control the quality of his stress responses during the day. . . . He would use controlled rhythmic breathing and refocus his attention elsewhere. He found that he felt less stressed overall."[68]

By reducing his stress, Frank was able to reduce his reliance on antibiotics and prescription retinoid creams. He began using his prescription remedies only at times when he knew he was under a lot of stress. Over the course of three months, his skin went from having regular, severe outbreaks of acne to mild, occasional outbreaks.

Alternative Medicine

Alternative medicine was once thought to be practiced only by herbalists, chiropractors, acupuncturists, naturopaths, and other non-Western practitioners. But in recent years alternative medical practices are becoming more accepted in the Western medical community. Some doctors and dermatologists, like Fried, are integrating alternative medicine into their practices.

Alternative practitioners believe that yoga or meditation can help acne sufferers by reducing stress levels.

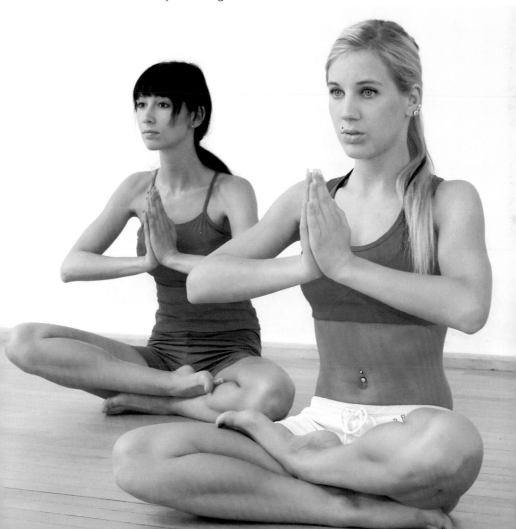

Alternative practitioners are doctors who take a nondrug approach to healing patients. They try to work with a patient to make changes to diet and lifestyle, emphasizing getting plenty of sleep, exercise, and good nutrition. They also emphasize using natural methods, such as yoga and meditation, to keep stress levels low. When medical intervention is needed, alternative practitioners tend to recommend natural remedies. They regard drug treatment as a last resort.

Stress

When acne is caused by stress, Western and alternative practitioners tend to agree on the best treatment—minimizing the stress. According to alternative health educator Billie Sahley, "Anger, depression, anxiety, and fear all cause measurable skin changes, including shifts in blood flow, moisture, and temperature."[69] But reducing stress can be very difficult. When stress is caused by a temporary problem, the solution may be to live with acne until the immediate source of stress—such as an exam, a relationship problem, or family issues—has passed. But for acne sufferers who face stressful situations every day as part of their work or family life, alternative practitioners may counsel that patients consider making changes to their lifestyles to reduce their overall stress levels.

Many alternative practitioners suggest that acne sufferers who have high stress levels spend less time taking care of other people, studying, or working and instead make more time to do things that they find relaxing. This could mean taking time to pursue a favorite hobby, such as gardening, exercising, or knitting. It could mean taking time to relax and get more sleep or taking time to meditate—sitting and focusing on breathing—once or twice a day. Or it could mean trying to make meaningful changes to their lives—getting counseling for family or relationship problems, leaving a dead-end job, moving to another part of the country, or deciding to pursue a dream, like going back to school or starting a new business.

In Frank's case dermatologist Richard Fried recommended guided imagery and short meditations in which Frank learned to relax by focusing on his breathing. Guided imagery is a process that patients can use to harness their minds to relax, let go of stress, and help their bodies to heal. "After 40 years of medical practice, I find guided imagery the easiest way for people to relax," explains family doctor Martin Rossman. "The simplest thing is to daydream yourself to a safe place of stresslessness." As a way of practicing guided imagery, Rossman encourages patients to relive, in their memory, the best experience of their lives. "They can do that in a fraction of a second," he says. "They can see what the day was like, what was said, the experience. It's multisensory. Imagery allows you to get that whole experience."[70]

Rossman explains that worry is also a form of guided imagery, but it is a negative form. When people worry all the time, they put their bodies into a perpetual state of alarm. "When the

Experts say that simple daydreaming can go a long way to help reduce teen stress.

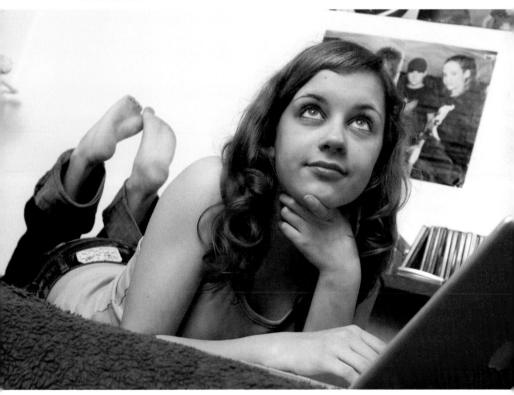

mind is full of worries," he says, "and you go over them day and night, your brain is constantly sending messages down through the autonomic nervous system to keep the body in an alarm state."[71] Staying in an alarm state means that the body releases the hormones adrenaline and cortisol into the blood stream. These hormones can stimulate the sebaceous glands and depress the immune system so that if pimples and cysts form, they will not heal very quickly.

Some massage therapists believe that patients can use the brain's ability to visualize—in other words, their imaginations —to increase blood flow on purpose to certain parts of the body, including the skin, helping those areas to heal. Other practitioners, including many Western psychologists and psychotherapists, simply believe that guided imagery is an easy way to help patients to relax. Relaxing gives acne patients a chance to let their bodies recover from surges of emotional hormones, giving the skin a chance to recover as well.

Acne and Depression Revisited

Western and alternative doctors alike are starting to believe that the link between acne and depression is malnutrition. Previously, it was thought that acne made people feel depressed and angry about how they looked. But now researchers have realized that the same nutrients that tend to be low in people with acne are also low in people who have depression and anxiety. In fact, these nutrients tend to be low in people with various kinds of mental disorders, including depression, anxiety, bipolar disorder, social anxiety disorder, and other mood disorders. These nutrients are the omega-3 fatty acids, zinc, selenium, chromium, and vitamin B_6.

Doctors are no longer certain that acne itself can cause depression and other disorders, or that the reverse is true. Instead, they suspect that malnutrition is the cause of both and can cause both acne and a mood disorder to arise in the same person.

Diet

No matter how much rest a patient gets, though, most alternative practitioners believe that acne will not clear until the patient begins to eat a well-balanced diet. To an alternative practitioner, eating a well-balanced diet means more than just following the guidelines on the U.S. Department of Agriculture's food pyramid. It means eating a diet that is based on whole foods, foods that have not been processed or have been processed only minimally. It also means eating a diet based on fruits and vegetables, with occasional small servings of whole grains. Meat, sugar, and dairy products, most alternative practitioners recommend, should be kept to a minimum in the diet.

Fruits and vegetables are important because they are food sources of vitamins and minerals that the body needs in order to repair its cells and grow new cells and tissues. Alternative practitioners have identified several nutrients that people with acne tend to be deficient in. Usually, people with acne need more foods containing omega-3 fatty acids, as well as adequate levels of important minerals such as zinc, magnesium, chromium, and selenium, and vitamins A, B, C, and E. Each nutrient serves important functions in the body. Each one is an anti-inflammatory, a substance that helps the body to reduce redness, swelling, and tenderness. Each of these nutrients is also a substance that studies show tends to be low in people with acne.

Why is nutrition so important for skin health? The omega-3 fatty acids are helpful for making sure that sebum contains enough linoleic acid to help skin cells slough off the sides of hair follicles efficiently, without getting stuck and forming comedones. Zinc and vitamin A are important in helping the body to grow new cells and repair its tissues, so they can help the skin to heal faster after an acne breakout. Zinc, the A and B vitamins, and vitamin C also provide support to the immune system. Having a healthy immune system can help the body to avoid bacterial infection, so pimples need not become as red and swollen as they otherwise might.

Acne patients may feel that they should be taking vitamin and mineral supplements. But studies show that people who do not have acne tend to eat more fruits and vegetables than people who seek treatment for acne. Alternative practitioners encourage their patients to do the same, in order to get their nutrients from whole foods. When foods are processed—cut, cooked, and powdered, for example—they lose some of their food value. Enzymes are destroyed in the cooking process. A fruit that has been juiced does not have as much fiber as a whole piece of fruit. "Sugar is a prime example," writes chiropractor Douglas Margel, "of how a whole food can be altered to its disadvantage. In its natural state, as sugar cane, it is a whole, complete food, full of healthy minerals and vitamins.

A steady diet containing lots of fruits and vegetables gives a person the vitamins and fatty acids that are essential to controlling acne.

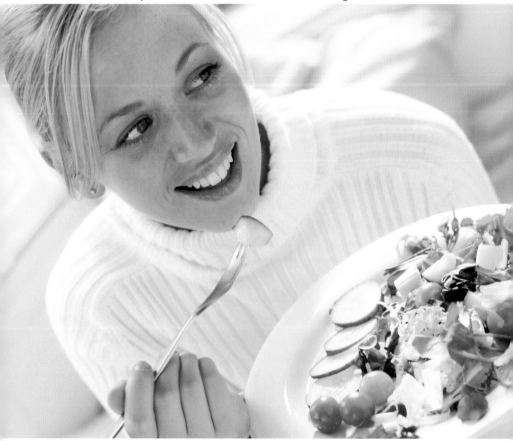

Yet, when refined, it is nothing but empty calories that are ultimately damaging to health."[72]

Food and Hormone Balance

In addition to providing the body with the nutrients it needs to grow, develop, and repair tissue by encouraging cells to reproduce, food also affects the balance of hormones in the body. Vitamin B$_6$ is thought to reduce the effects of testosterone on the body. The phytochemicals in soybeans have the effect of reducing the amount of testosterone and other androgens in the blood, so the androgen receptors in the sebaceous glands are less likely to become overstimulated. Lycopene, a substance that forms in cooked tomatoes, also reduces testosterone in the blood. Raw almonds can help keep blood sugar levels stable and are connected with stable levels of insulin in the blood. High-fiber meals also tend to hold down the levels of testosterone in the blood. Green tea helps to keep hormone levels stable.

Just as some foods can help to balance and control hormones, however, other foods can cause hormones to surge out of control. Sugar, meat, dairy products, and vegetable oils are some of the worst offenders. "What you eat affects your hormones," warns acne specialist Elaine Mummery, who started her own acne clinic in Glasgow, Scotland. Eating a lot of meat and grains causes the levels of cortisol in the blood to climb, while eating a lot of sugar and starch can cause insulin to spike. "If you tend to eat refined foods—white bread, sugary drinks, fast food—your body digests it very quickly," Mummery explains. "Because of that it raises your blood sugar levels and to correct that your body produces insulin. That insulin raises your testosterone levels and that produces sebum, which clogs your pores and causes acne."[73]

Skin Diabetes

In the early part of the twentieth century, dermatologists were so concerned about blood sugar spikes and insulin surges that they often referred to acne as "skin diabetes" or "cutaneous diabetes." Patients with acne, they found, might not have particularly high levels of sugar or insulin in their blood. Instead, acne patients had high levels of sugar in their skin. One study showed that after a person eats a sugary snack, sugar levels in the skin remain elevated for 226 minutes.

Many alternative practitioners, like Mummery, have come to believe that sugar, because of the insulin surges that it causes, is one of the worst foods you can eat when it comes to your skin's health. Dermatologists used to disagree. For most of the latter half of the twentieth century, dermatologists claimed that there was no connection between diet and acne. In recent years though, dermatologists such as Richard Fried have come to believe that patients should try to avoid any foods that they consider to be personal triggers for their acne. Fried advocates that patients keep a journal in which they record everything they ate each day, how much exercise they got, what they wore, what products they used on their skin, and how their acne was that day. This way patients may be able to identify their personal triggers. Anecdotally, dermatologists say that patients often identify sugar as a trigger.

In 2007 Australian researchers decided to study this issue. They were interested in how the position of a food on the glycemic index might affect hormone levels. Foods that are low on the glycemic index (often referred to as low-GI foods) are foods that are digested slowly. They do not cause any sudden spikes in blood sugar. Peanuts, grapefruit, and apples are low-GI foods. High-GI foods, on the other hand, are digested very quickly. They cause blood sugar levels to spike quickly and sometimes blood sugar will remain high for several hours. Table sugar is a high-GI food, but so are many foods that do not taste sweet, such as baked potatoes, white bread, and white rice.

The Australian researchers had their study subjects focus on eating foods that contained plenty of protein but were low on the glycemic index. After three months they noticed that blood insulin levels had dropped dramatically in the low-GI group, as compared to the control group (the group that ate foods that were high on the GI scale). At the same time the patients in the low-GI group were pleased to discover that their faces were clearing up and that they were losing weight. Losing weight af-

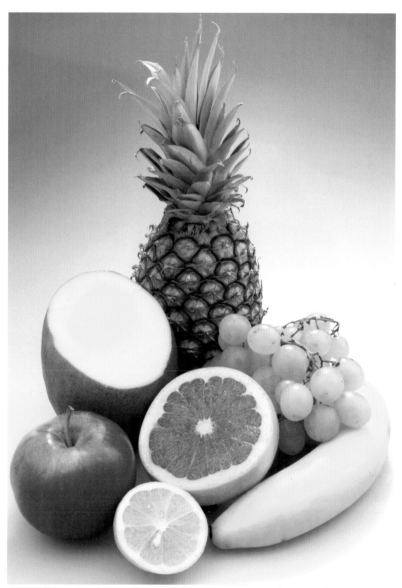

One of the simplest, most natural ways to control acne is by incorporating plenty of fresh fruit into the diet.

fected their acne too, because in women, fat cells produce cortisol and androgens. Androgens bind with androgen receptors in the sebaceous glands, causing an increase in sebum production and an increase in acne.

Smoker's Acne

There is one lifestyle change that all dermatologists and alternative practitioners agree will improve acne: quitting smoking. A 2007 study showed that nearly half of adults who smoke have acne. Most get noninflammatory acne (NIA). It consists primarily of whiteheads, blackheads, and small cysts in the area around the mouth and chin. The cysts can range from mild to moderate but do not usually get very red.

About three quarters of people who have NIA smoke. Among people who have severe NIA, more than 80 percent are smokers, and the rest had been exposed to secondhand smoke. Dermatologists are thinking of changing the name of NIA to "smoker's acne."

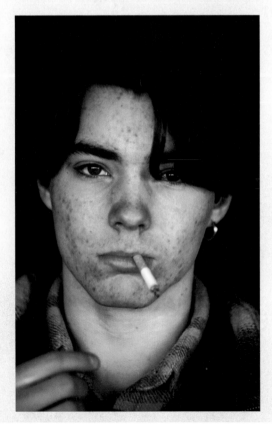

Smoking can cause whiteheads, blackheads, and small cysts around the mouth.

Traditionally, Western doctors and alternative practitioners have viewed each other with a great deal of skepticism. However, Western dermatologists are learning more about the importance of nutrition, while alternative practitioners are using scientific tests and clinical trials to help them demonstrate the value of alternative strategies for producing good health. In some cases dermatologists and alternative practitioners are beginning to work as partners. In the future it is possible that Western and alternative medicine may share office space so that Western and alternative practitioners can refer patients to each other. (In some medical centers, such as Alternative Medical Integration of Illinois, they already do.) They may consult each other on tough cases. Many medical doctors and alternative practitioners feel sure that they will be consulting each other regularly and sharing information, no matter what the future of medicine may hold.

CHAPTER SIX

The Future of Acne Treatment

"**I**'m under house arrest," writes longtime acne sufferer Leslie Inglis. "My blinds are closed and I'm shackled to my couch with ice packs on my face."[74] Inglis had just finished the fourth of four sessions using an unusual new acne treatment—photodynamic, or blue-light, therapy.

Photodynamic Acne Treatment

Photodynamic treatment (PDT) is a new therapy that uses light to treat many different kinds of disorders, ranging from cancer to age-related blindness. When it is used to treat acne, PDT is often called blue-light therapy, because it uses the blue part of the light spectrum. Blue light can temporarily sterilize the skin, killing bacteria and healing mild to moderate breakouts. It works well for healing papules, pustules, and some nodules, but it cannot heal comedones or cysts. Consequently, dermatologists usually prescribe a topical ointment or cream in addition to PDT.

PDT sessions take time. Many patients have PDT for about fifteen minutes at a time, twice a week, for four weeks or more. During PDT, the patient must first lie down. Then a nurse cleans the patient's face with alcohol or acetone. Some patients also have microdermabrasion, a process similar to dermabrasion, in which tiny, rough grains are used to rub off the top layer of skin. Then a photosensitizing drug—a drug that makes the skin more sensitive to light—is applied. The skin is dried, and after a short wait (thirty to sixty minutes), the patient sits in front of a blue light. "It's kind of like a tanning booth on your face,"[75] explains Pauline Muzyka, a New York dental assistant who went through PDT.

While being exposed to the light source used in PDT, the patient may feel warmth, tingling, or even a burning sensation. "The process . . . feels like hundreds of tiny rubber bands snapping at your face (unpleasant, but not insanely painful),"[76]

A laser is used in photodynamic acne therapy. It produces a blue light that temporarily sterilizes the skin, killing bacteria and healing mild acne outbreaks.

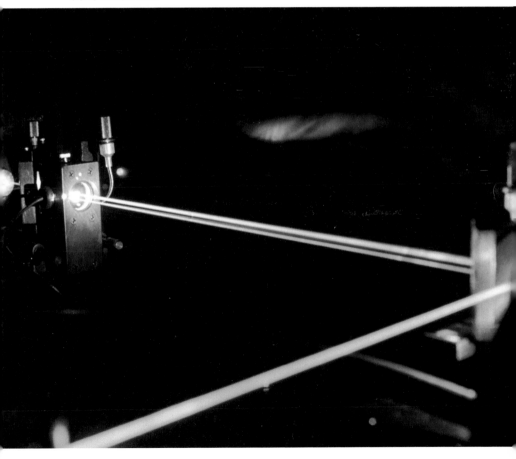

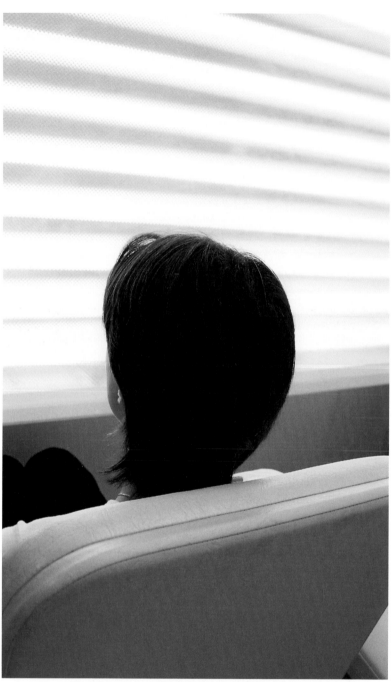

A woman undergoes photodynamic treatment. Although the treatments take time and are expensive, they are effective.

wrote PDT patient Andrea Lavinthal a few weeks after her treatment. Patients can hold a fan during the light application and use it to cool off their skin as needed.

After PDT the skin remains unusually sensitive to light for several days. Patients who receive PDT must be prepared to protect their skin rigorously from the sun for up to three days after each treatment. "I was given strict orders to avoid the sun for a few days," remembers Lavinthal. "When I did leave my apartment, I had to wear a hat, sunglasses, and a scarf. . . . Plus I was forbidden to wash or moisturize my face for four whole days . . . my skin was red, raw, and drier than the Sahara."[77]

PDT is expensive, ranging from $250 to $600 per session. A patient may need as many as eight sessions. And some patients find the treatment unpleasant. But it does produce good results for many acne sufferers. One study showed a 60 percent reduction in the number of pimples on patients' skin after eight PDT sessions. The sebaceous glands shrink during PDT, and sebum production remains low for at least six months after the treatment. Lavinthal says that a month afterward, she felt her treatment was worth it—her acne was gone, her scars were much less noticeable, and she felt she could skip wearing makeup sometimes. However, some dermatologists are still skeptical. Miami dermatologist Alicia Barba says that PDT may help shrink sebaceous glands temporarily. But, she says, it is still not as effective as Accutane (isotretinoin). "What Accutane does is pretty miraculous," says Barba. "I do not think we're there yet with photodynamic therapy."[78]

Lasers

Laser therapy is another new way to use light to treat acne. Laser light, though, is much higher in intensity than the blue light used for PDT. Laser light is pure, high-energy light. It is focused, meaning that the light is all one wavelength and all one frequency, and the crests and troughs of the waves travel together. Laser light is the only kind of light that has waves that are all the same and travel in sync with each other. This property of laser light is what makes it useful to doctors. Surgeons can use lasers to do precision surgery—they can remove tissue that is unwanted without harming any of the surrounding tissue. Lasers can be used to cut through tissue without causing too much bleeding, explains Richard Felton, a medical device reviewer for the FDA. They can also be used to cause blood and tissue to coagulate, or stop bleeding. "That's something a knife can't do,"[79] Felton points out. Lasers are so precise that they can even be used to operate on the human eye.

Lasers can be helpful for treating inflammatory acne, such as papules and pustules. Studies show that laser light can greatly reduce the number of acne lesions that a patient has even after just one treatment. After four such treatments the number of lesions drops even more dramatically. The improvements to the skin remain for at least six months.

Although lasers can be very effective for treating acne and minimizing the appearance of scars, the procedure is not an easy one to go through. Lasers are used to remove the epidermis from the skin. Doctors numb the skin with local anesthetics first, and they give the patient a sedative to help him or her to relax. But it may still be an uncomfortable process. South Carolina teacher Tonya Carter described it as "a little sting, like a rubber band prick at you."[80] Carter said that each treatment left her with a series of tiny red dots on her face. Patients who have general resurfacing of their entire faces, though, are left looking and feeling as though they have been badly sunburned. Right after laser treatment, the skin is raw, sore, and oozy. It may also blister. As it begins to heal and new skin forms, it may tingle, burn, or itch. The face must be kept covered and moist for the first few days, and patients must avoid direct sunlight for the next year.

It takes about a month to recover from laser resurfacing, but patients are often very pleased with the results. After six such treatments, Carter said, her acne was "pretty much wiped out."[81]

Lasers have also become a safe, standard way to treat acne scarring, according to Michael Goldman of the American Academy of Dermatologists. He states: "The . . . laser . . . is an excellent new method for treating acne scars because it works for all skin types—from very dark to very light—and with no downtime. Until now, many of the other acne scar treatments produced a wound that may have required weeks to heal. Since this new laser therapy is noninvasive, the patient does not require anesthesia and the procedure is not a painful one."[82] Some patients have individual scars treated with lasers. Small surface scars can be smoothed out with lasers. Deep scars can be removed and stitched together, or a skin graft can be used to fill the space left when the scar is removed.

Many patients, though, are choosing to have laser resurfacing of the entire face. Laser resurfacing is a technique that doctors discovered accidentally, while using lasers to repair acne scars. After a scar was repaired, surgeons decided to try resurfacing the skin around the scar, to make the scar less visible. When they did so, they found that wrinkles and small imperfections in the skin's

---

Stopping Acne with Chocolate

Many people who suffer from acne blame chocolate, but dermatologists say there is no connection between chocolate and acne. In 2007 though, manufacturers began to produce chocolate bars packed with ingredients that are intended to stop acne from forming. The bars are made of 72 percent raw cacao, unlike ordinary milk chocolate, which has sugar as its primary ingredient. Cacao is a good source of magnesium, which is thought to be an important mineral for preventing acne. The bars also contain walnut-husk extract (another magnesium source), as well as pomegranate extract and green tea extract (for their anti-inflammatory properties).

The manufacturers of the new bars—Borba Chocolate Clarifying Bar and Acne Care chocolate bars—are hopeful. Dermatologists though, are skeptical. "It's a 'walletectomy,'" says dermatologist James Spencer of St. Petersburg, Florida. "You can get the same benefit from a Flintstones chewable [vitamin]."

Quoted in Betsy Streisand, "Selling the Idea That You Are What You Eat," *US News & World Report*, April 22, 2007. www.usnews.com/usnews/biztech/articles/0704 22/30eespotlight.htm.

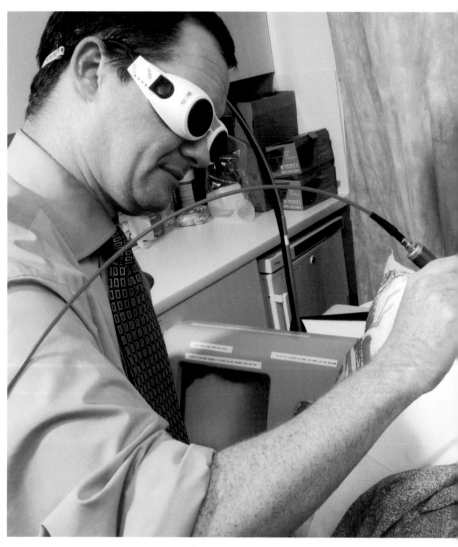

surface were greatly diminished. Now laser resurfacing is offered as a cosmetic procedure for the entire face. Not only can it make scars less visible, it can also reduce wrinkles, sun damage, freckles, and damage caused by smoking. "Resurfacing is very appealing to people," says Indianapolis plastic surgeon Stephen Perkins, "because it is a way of refreshing the skin's surface and getting a new layer of non-sun-damaged and more youthful skin."[83]

Washington, D.C., laser surgeon Tina Alster agrees, but she warns that this kind of procedure is not right for everyone.

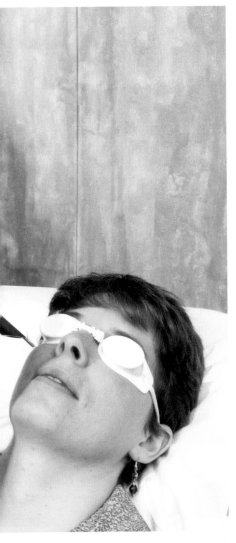

A doctor uses a laser to remove acne-related scar tissue from a young woman's face.

"This is not easy-in, easy-out surgery," she cautions. "Patients have to realize that there will be bruising and swelling and they will be holed up in the house for seven to ten days. They will have a crusty, oozy, bruised, scabbed, raw-appearing face."[84]

Probiotic Lotion

Patients who prefer a gentler approach to acne treatment may decide that they prefer the new probiotic lotions that are being developed. Probiotic lotions are lotions that include bacteria, such as *Lactobacillus* that are known to be beneficial to the skin. These bacteria, unlike *P. acnes*, the bacterium that causes acne, can restore the skin's natural bacterial balance. They compete with *P. acnes* and make it hard for *P. acnes* to get entrenched in the hair follicles. Since probiotic bacteria do not kill *P. acnes* directly, they do not cause the development of probiotic resistance—unlike antibiotic acne remedies, which can promote the development of antibiotic-resistant bacteria.

Probiotic creams are not a drug, so they do not have to be prescribed by a doctor. Acne sufferers can go to a pharmacy to buy the creams and apply them as part of their own self-care at home. Researchers are not sure yet how effective the probiotic

Acne Zappers

Several manufacturers have started producing handheld, portable electronic devices that acne sufferers can use in place of over-the-counter creams to combat occasional acne break-outs. The Zeno and Thermaclear are handheld heaters, meant to warm a pimple for a short time in order to kill bacteria and improve the body's anti-inflammatory response. The Zeno heats the skin to about 120°F (49°C) and keeps it at that temperature for about two and a half minutes. Thermaclear heats the skin much more, to 212°F (100°C), but for a much shorter time, two and a half seconds. Thermaclear is faster, but some users say it hurts.

Some acne sufferers also like to use the NuFace, a portable, handheld device that "zaps" pimples with an electrical current. The NuFace is meant to be more like a facial—users apply conductivity gel and then roll the NuFace all over the face, avoiding the eyes. The NuFace is meant for all kinds of facial irregularities, including wrinkles, acne, and rosacea.

These three devices are expensive, however (from $100 to $225 per device), and dermatologists are skeptical. Studies show that the Zeno and Thermaclear work if they are applied quickly, at the first sign of a pimple. NuFace has been shown to be effective in reducing wrinkles, but it is not yet clear whether it works well for acne. Some dermatologists point out that antibiotics work just as well and are faster to apply.

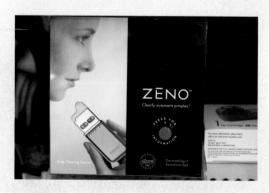

The Zeno acne clearing device is just one of many "acne zappers" on the market.

creams are at treating acne, but they are optimistic because studies have shown that probiotic creams can improve itching and eczema. Some dermatologists though, are still skeptical. "Until more microbiological studies can prove it," commented British doctor Nick Lowe, "I'll continue eating my yoghurt rather than smearing it on my face."[85]

Although dermatologists continue to develop new methods of treating acne, they still use the old methods, too. Most dermatologists feel strongly that tools such as retinoids and antibiotics will always be necessary to clear up really stubborn cases of acne. The newer methods though, give them something else they can try when a patient has a very stubborn case of acne or does not want to try drug treatments. Rather than replacing the old methods of diagnosis and treatment, new twenty-first-century methods will add to the dermatological repertoire, giving patients and doctors the choices and the hope that they urgently need.

Notes

Introduction: A Common Problem

1. Quoted in Ann-Marie Schiro, "Patterns," *New York Times*, December 15, 1992.
2. Quoted in *Mail*, "Keira Takes Kate's Crown," March 5, 2006, p. 9.
3. Vail Reese, "'Zits Are the Pitts.' What Makes Jolie Not Jolly?" Skinema. www.skinema.com/Act1Acne.html.
4. Quoted in Katie Rodan, Kathy Fields, and Vanessa Williams, *Unblemished*. New York: Simon & Schuster, 2004, p. 71.
5. Quoted in Daniel Shorn, "Adult Acne Treatments Go High Tech," CBS News, December 26, 2005. www.cbsnews.com/stories/2005/12/26/earlyshow/health/main1165729.shtml.
6. Quoted in *Toronto Star*, "Acne Is a Painful Battle," April 17, 2003. p. H04.
7. Quoted in Mary Brophy Marcus, "Acne Leaves Emotional Marks," *USA Today*, February 12, 2007, p. 07d.
8. Quoted in Marcus, "Acne Leaves Emotional Marks."
9. Quoted in Samantha Critchell, "New Treatments Popping Up for Adults with Acne," *Toronto Star*, March 7, 2008, p. L03.
10. Mark Morford, "That Is Not Really Cameron Diaz," *San Francisco Chronicle*. May 23, 2008. www.sfgate.com/cgi-bin/article.cgi?f=/g/a/2008/05/23/notes052308.DTL.
11. *Mail*, "Keira Takes Kate's Crown," p. 9.

Chapter One: What Happens During an Acne Breakout?

12. Quoted in *Toronto Star*, "Acne Is a Painful Battle." p. H04.
13. Quoted in Marcus, "Acne Leaves Emotional Marks."
14. Quoted in Lydia Preston and Tina Alster, *Breaking Out*. New York: Simon & Schuster, 2004, p. 31.
15. Vanessa Williams, "A Proactiv Solution Success Story," Proactiv. www.proactiv.com/celebrity/vanessa-williams.php.

16. Quoted in Rodan, Fields, and Williams, *Unblemished*, p. 66.
17. Quoted in Rodan, Fields, and Williams, *Unblemished*, p. 74.
18. Serena Williams, "A Proactiv Solution Success Story," Proactiv. www.proactiv.com/celebrity/serena-williams.php.
19. Quoted in Rodan, Fields, and Williams, *Unblemished*, p. 74.

Chapter Two: Causes of Acne

20. Jennifer Berry, "A Proactiv Solution Success Story," Proactiv. www.proactiv.com/celebrity/jennifer-berry.php.
21. Berry, "A Proactiv Solution Success Story."
22. Chrishell Stause, "A Proactiv Solution Success Story," Proactiv. www.proactiv.com/celebrity/chrishell-stause.php.
23. Quoted in American Academy of Dermatologists, "Millions of Women Facing Adult Acne," July 30, 2004. www.aad .org/media/background/news/Releases/Millions_of_Women _Facing_Adult_Acne.
24. Quoted in Natasha Singer, "Skin Deep: Why Should Kids Have All the Acne?" *New York Times*, October 18, 2007. http://query.nytimes.com/gst/fullpage.html?res=9C05EF DF133AF93BA25753C1A9619C8B63&sec=&spon=&&scp=11 4&sq=acne&st=cse.
25. American Academy of Dermatologists, "Millions of Women Facing Adult Acne."
26. Jennifer Love Hewitt, "A Proactiv Solution Success Story," Proactiv. www.proactiv.com/celebrity/jennifer-love-hewitt.php.
27. Jessica Simpson, "A Proactiv Solution Success Story," Proactiv. www.proactiv.com/celebrity/jessica-simpson.php.
28. Quoted in *USA Today (Society for the Advancement of Education)*, "Mites Might Cause Mighty Problems," February 2004, p. 14.
29. Quoted in *USA Today (Society for the Advancement of Education)*, "Mites Might Cause Mighty Problems," p. 14.
30. Quoted in *USA Today (Society for the Advancement of Education)*, "Mites Might Cause Mighty Problems," p. 14.
31. Quoted in Sharon Snider, "Acne: Taming That Age-Old Adolescent Affliction," *FDA Consumer*, October 1990, p. 16.

Chapter Three: Self-Treatment of Acne

32. Quoted in Preston and Alster, *Breaking Out*, p. 43.

33. Quoted in Snider, "Acne," p. 16.
34. Richard Fried, *Healing Adult Acne*. Oakland, CA: New Harbinger, 2005, p. 29.
35. Quoted in Preston and Alster, *Breaking Out*, p. 62.
36. Quoted in Preston and Alster, *Breaking Out*, p. 62.
37. Quoted in Preston and Alster, *Breaking Out*, p. 64.
38. Quoted in Rene Brooks Catacalos, "Handle with Care: Shalea Walker Goes Skin Deep," *Black Enterprise*, November 2006, p. 161.
39. Quoted in Preston and Alster, *Breaking Out*, p. 64.
40. Quoted in Preston and Alster, *Breaking Out*, p. 64.
41. Quoted in Catacalos, "Handle with Care," p. 161.
42. Quoted in American Academy of Dermatologists, "Millions of Women Facing Adult Acne."
43. Quoted in American Academy of Dermatologists, "Millions of Women Facing Adult Acne."
44. Quoted in Preston and Alster, *Breaking Out*, p. 46.
45. Quoted in Singer, "Skin Deep."
46. Quoted in Preston and Alster, *Breaking Out*, p. 62.
47. Quoted in Preston and Alster, *Breaking Out*, p. 61.
48. Quoted in Preston and Alster, *Breaking Out*, p. 61.
49. Quoted in Singer, "Skin Deep."

Chapter Four: Medical Treatment for Acne

50. Quoted in Lindsay Fergus, "Acne Got Me in a Spot of Bother," *Mirror*, October 2, 2006, p. 19.
51. Quoted in Paul Swiech, "Acne Solutions," *Pantagraph*, September 15, 2006. http://search.ebscohost.com/login.aspx?direct=direct=true&db=nfh&AN=2W62W61157203880&site=ehost-live.
52. Fried, *Healing Adult Acne*, p. 23.
53. Fried, *Healing Adult Acne*, p. 55.
54. Quoted in Sally Wadyka, "The Thing About Retin-A: It Works," *New York Times*, November 30, 2006. www.nytimes.com/2006/11/30/fashion/30skin.html?scp=11&sq=retin-A%20acne&st=cse.
55. Quoted in Stause, "A Proactiv Solution Success Story."
56. Fried, *Healing Adult Acne*, p. 51.

57. Quoted in *Toronto Star*, "Acne Is a Painful Battle," p. H04.
58. Quoted in John Jesitus, "Isotretinoin and Suicide: Epidemiological Study Shows No Association," *Dermatology Times*, April 30, 2009. http://dermatologytimes.modernmedicine .com/dermatologytimes/Acne/Isotretinoin-and-suicide-Epi demiological-studysho/ArticleStandard/Article/detail/ 595931?ref=25.
59. Quoted in Bonnie Estridge, "I Would Dread Boys Running Their Hands over My Body," *Daily Mail*, April 2, 1996, p. 38.
60. Quoted in Critchell, "New Treatments Popping Up for Adults with Acne," p. L03.
61. Quoted in Camilla Herrera, "About Face: Expert Zaps Acne Myths, Offers Treatment Tips," *Stamford Advocate*, November 14, 2006. http://search.ebscohost.com/login.aspx?direct =true& db=nfh&AN=2W62W6532195690&site=ehost-live.
62. Quoted in American Academy of Dermatologists, "Millions of Women Facing Adult Acne." www.aad.org/media/background/ news/Releases/Millions_of_Women_Facing_Adult_Acne/.
63. Quoted in *Journal of Drugs in Dermatology*, "Office-Based Procedure," July 1, 2004. www.accessmylibrary.com/coms2/ summary_0286-3910405_ITM.
64. Quoted in *Journal of Drugs in Dermatology*, "Office-Based Procedure."
65. Quoted in Marcus, "Acne Leaves Emotional Marks," p. 07d.
66. Fried, *Healing Adult Acne*, p. 86.
67. Quoted in Marcus, "Acne Leaves Emotional Marks," p. 07d.

Chapter Five: Alternative Treatments for Acne

68. Fried, *Healing Adult Acne*, p. 42.
69. Billie Sahley, "Acne and Other Skin Problems," *MMRC Health Educator Reports*, 2008, pp. 1–2.
70. Quoted in Karrie Osborn, "Guided Imagery and Massage," *Massage and Bodywork*, May/June 2008. www.massagether apy.com/articles/index.php/article_id/1568/Guided-Im agery-and-Massage.
71. Quoted in Osborn, "Guided Imagery and Massage."
72. Quoted in Douglas Margel, *The Nutrient-Dense Eating*

Plan. Laguna Beach, CA: Basic Health, 2005, p. 71.

73. Quoted in Sarah Swain, "Elaine Out to Help You Get Spotless: Mum Writes a Book to Help End Misery of Acne," *Evening Times* (Glasgow, Scotland), June 2, 2009, p. 20.

Chapter Six: The Future of Acne Treatment

74. Inglis, Leslie. "Acne Sufferer Finally Sees the Light," *Toronto Star*, June 23, 2005, p. E01.

75. Quoted in Laurel Geraghty, "Light or Heat Treatments as Alternatives to Drug," *New York Times*, January 12, 2006. www.nytimes.com/2006/01/12/fashion/thursdaystyles/12 sside.html?scp=1&sq=photodynamic%20therapy%20acne& st=cse.

76. Andrea Lavinthal, "The Crazy Thing I Did for Clear Skin," *Cosmopolitan*, March 18, 2009. www.cosmopolitan.com/ hairstyles-beauty/beauty-blog/clear-skin-treatment?click= main_sr.

77. Lavinthal, "The Crazy Thing I Did for Clear Skin."

78. Quoted in Marcus, "Acne Leaves Emotional Marks," p. 07d.

79. Quoted in Alexandra Greeley, "Cosmetic Laser Surgery," *FDA Consumer*, May 2000, p. 34.

80. Quoted in Geraghty, "Light or Heat Treatments as Alternatives to Drug."

81. Quoted in Geraghty, "Light or Heat Treatments as Alternatives to Drug."

82. Quoted in *Health and Medicine Net*, "Laser Treatment Helps Heal the Physical and Emotional Scars of Acne," 2001. www.obgyn.net/newsrx/general_health-Dermatology-20010827-18.asp.

83. Quoted in Greeley, "Cosmetic Laser Surgery," p. 34.

84. Quoted in Greeley, "Cosmetic Laser Surgery," p. 34.

85. Quoted in Claire Coleman, "Probiotic Beauty," *Mail Online*, April 20, 2009. http://www.dailymail.co.uk/femail/article-11 71940/Probiotic-beauty-Theyre-bugs-boost-digestion--clean-skin.html.

Glossary

alternative medicine: A nondrug approach to healing, emphasizing lifestyle changes, such as a healthy diet, exercise, and rest and using natural remedies when medical intervention is needed.

androgens: Hormones that are predominantly found in men, such as testosterone.

antibiotics: Drugs that kill bacteria.

benzoyl peroxide: An antibacterial drug that is applied to the surface of the skin.

chemical peel: A chemical solution used to cause the skin's top layer to separate from the rest of the skin and peel off.

comedo: A plug made of dead epidermal skin cells.

comedo extraction: The process of removing or draining the contents of a blackhead, whitehead, or cyst.

comedone: A blemish formed when a hair follicle is blocked by a comedo.

dermabrasion: The process of mechanically rubbing off or sanding away the top layer of skin.

dermatologist: A doctor specializing in the diagnosis and treatment of skin disorders.

dermis: The middle layer of the skin.

epidermis: The outer layer of the skin.

exfoliant: An ingredient that works well for removing dead skin cells and dirt from the surface of the skin.

hair follicle: A small sac in the skin, out of which a hair can grow.

hormones: Chemicals produced by the body's glands and released as a signal to tell cells and tissues in another part of the body to do something.

inflammation: Redness and swelling.

isotretinoin: Also called Accutane, this is the strongest of the retinoid drugs.

laser therapy: The use of a high-energy, focused laser light to take off the top layer of skin so that a new, smoother layer can form in its place.

oral contraceptives: Hormones that can prevent pregnancy and hormonally caused acne in many women.

over-the-counter remedy: A medicine that can be purchased without a prescription.

P. acnes: A bacterium that lives deep in the skin and infects pimples.

photodynamic treatment (PDT): Therapy that uses light to cure disorders; also called blue-light therapy.

probiotic lotion: A lotion that contains living bacteria and is used to bring the skin's ecosystem back into balance.

puberty: A developmental stage in which the hypothalamus and pituitary glands release hormones governing sexual development.

retinoids: Drugs that are derived from vitamin A.

salicylic acid: An exfoliant and anti-inflammatory drug that can be applied to the surface of the skin.

sebaceous glands: Glands that produce sebum, or oil.

subcutaneous tissue: The deepest layer of skin, containing the fat that cushions the body against bumps and falls.

Organizations to Contact

American Academy of Dermatology
1350 I St. NW, Ste. 180
Washington, DC 20005-3305
phone: (202) 842-3555
fax: (202) 842-4355
Web site: www.aad.org

The American Academy of Dermatology represents nearly all dermatologists in the United States. The academy publishes several magazines and journals, offers referrals to dermatologists, produces press releases and fact sheets, advocates on behalf of dermatologists when federal and state legislation related to skin care is being considered, and maintains a separate section of its Web site (www.skincarephysicians.com/acne net/index.html) devoted to educating the public about acne.

National Institute of Arthritis and Musculoskeletal and Skin Diseases
1 AMS Circle
Bethesda, MD 20892-3675
phone: (301) 495-4484
fax: (301) 718-6366
Web site: www.niams.nih.gov/Health_Info/Acne/default.asp

The National Institute of Arthritis and Musculoskeletal and Skin Diseases is a department of the National Institutes of Health, which is part of the U.S. Department of Health and Human Services. The Web site includes a pamphlet updated with the most recent research on acne and other skin diseases. There are links to journal articles and news releases related to acne, as well as information about clinical trials that are currently in progress or being organized. There is also a link to a Spanish version of the entire Web site.

For Further Reading

Books

Alan Logan and Valori Treloar, *The Clear Skin Diet*. Nashville, TN: Cumberland House, 2007. An overview of dietary and naturopathic approaches to treating acne, written by a member of Harvard Medical School's Mind/Body Medical Institute.

Robert Norman, *The Woman Who Lost Her Skin and Other Dermatological Tales*. New York and Oxford: Routledge, 2004. Includes one chapter devoted to acne and other chapters related to other skin disorders. The acne chapter describes the skin as an ecosystem and explains what organisms normally reside in and on the skin: bacteria, mites, viruses, and fungi.

Lydia Preston and Tina Alster, *Breaking Out*. New York: Simon & Schuster, 2004. Includes a detailed explanation of what happens in a breakout, how hormones affect the process of acne development, and over-the-counter and prescription remedies for acne.

Katie Rodan, Kathy Fields, and Vanessa Williams, *Unblemished*. New York: Simon & Schuster, 2004. A book by the dermatologists who developed Proactiv, a commonly used over-the-counter acne remedy. Explains the role of bacteria in acne development and includes information about new techniques for treating acne, such as light therapy.

Guy Webster and Anthony Rawlings, *Acne and Its Therapy*. Boca Raton, FL: CRC, 2007. An anthology of scientific and detailed articles on different aspects of acne, such as the formation of comedones, retinoid treatment, light therapy, and the use of benzoyl peroxide and salicylic acid.

Web Sites

"Acne," KidsHealth, Nemours (http://kidshealth.org/kid/grow/ body_stuff/acne.html). A website on acne intended for kids. Includes basic explanation of how acne forms and links to related topics, such as puberty, menstruation, acne myths, and skin care.

American Academy of Dermatology, Acne.net (www.skin carephysicians.com/acnenet/). An educational Web site provided by the American Academy of Dermatology. Includes pages on what acne is and how it develops, treatment, scarring, myths, social impact, and when to see a dermatologist. Also includes a tool for finding a dermatologist in a particular geographic area.

"Skin Care: Top 5 Habits for Healthy Skin," Mayo Clinic (www.mayoclinic.com/health/skin-care/SN00003). The Mayo Clinic's page on basic skin care, with tips for preventing skin disorders ranging from acne to skin cancer. Includes links to pages on related topics, such as dry skin, age spots, and sunscreen.

"Under the Microscope," BAM! Body and Mind, Centers for Disease Control and Prevention (www.bam.gov/sub _yourbody/yourbody_bodysmartz_microscope.html). A summary for preteens of how acne forms, myths about acne, and how to treat acne. Focuses on the connection between acne and puberty.

Index

Picture Credits

About the Author

Bonnie Juettner is a writer and editor of children's reference books. She frequently writes about science and health-related topics. Her other books for the Diseases and Disorders series include *Skin Cancer* and *Thyroid Disorders*.